CUPPING THERAPY

FOR MUSCLES AND JOINTS

An Easy-to-Understand Guide for Relieving Pain,
Reducing Inflammation and Healing Injury

KENNETH CHOI

ULYSSES PRESS

Published in the United States by:
Ulysses Press
P.O. Box 3440
Berkeley, CA 94703
www.ulyssespress.com

Printed in the United States
10 9 8 7 6 5 4 3 2 1

ISBN: 978-1-64604-229-6
Library of Congress Control Number: 2018930755

Acquisitions editor: Bridget Thoreson
Managing editor: Claire Chun
Project editor: Shayna Keyles
Editor: Renee Rutledge
Proofreader: Shayna Keyles
Indexer: Sayre Van Young
Front cover design: Malea Clark-Nicholson
Interior design and layout: what!design @ whatweb.com
Cover artwork: © Andrey_Popov/shutterstock.com
Interior artwork: page 34 © Peter Hermes Furian/shutterstock.com; page 35 © Designua/
    shutterstock.com; page 36 © Stihi/shutterstock.com

CONTENTS

INTRODUCTION

Just a few decades ago, cupping was almost unheard of in North America. It was not a very popular treatment, and when people got it done, they would hide what they considered unsightly cupping marks to avoid drawing attention to them. However, in recent years, cupping has experienced a huge surge in popularity and public figures have been seen adorning cupping marks almost as a fashion statement.

The most highly covered story of cupping was when the most decorated Olympian of all time, Michael Phelps, with 28 Olympic medals (23 of them gold), was seen with cupping marks on his right shoulder and legs during the 2016 Olympics in Rio de Janeiro. The internet blew up with everyone talking about it, and the media raced to uncover the mysterious "red marks" on his body, which brought cupping into public consciousness. Phelps publicly endorsed cupping as a good way to recover and relieve tired or sore muscles, posting Instagram photos of the treatment and talking about it during interviews. Since then, more and more athletes, including US Olympic gymnast Alex Naddour, 12-time Olympic medalist Natalie Coughlin, and NBA All-Star and MVP Stephen Curry, have had cupping therapy done, hoping it will give them an edge over their competitors.

Cupping has also been popular in Hollywood, with celebrities showing up to red carpet events and press conferences with cupping marks. Notable celebrities that have shown them off include Jennifer Aniston, Gwyneth Paltrow, Kaley Cuoco, Victoria Beckham, and Justin Bieber. Cupping has also been the subject of conversation on *The Ellen DeGeneres Show*, where Nicole Richie shared a picture of her father, legendary singer Lionel Richie, getting cupping done.

Thanks to these athletes and celebrities, cupping has become very trendy and more people are increasingly open to it. It has also introduced people to the world of Traditional Chinese Medicine (TCM), where cupping is still a primary modality used to stop pain and treat injuries, internal diseases, gynecological problems, and dermatological problems.

In this book, I will talk about what cupping is, how it works, and how to use cupping to treat sports injuries, pain on specific areas of the body, and various diseases, including digestive problems, gynecological problems, infections, respiratory disorders, skin conditions, and psychological or mental issues like stress and insomnia. I will also cover different types of cupping sets, cupping techniques, and cupping safety.

CHAPTER 1

WHAT IS CUPPING THERAPY?

Cupping therapy is a Traditional Chinese Medicine therapy that has been used for more than 3,000 years. It involves using special cups to apply suction over the skin of an affected area. Many different methods are used to produce a vacuum inside the cup to create this suction, from heating the cup to using a mechanical pump to just using the mouth to suck the air out. The negative pressure created in the cup causes the skin to draw upward into the cup. The cups are then left in place or moved around the skin to improve the blood circulation in the area, rid the body of toxins, improve general well-being, and help with many different ailments, including pain, inflammation, infections, and snake and insect bites.

HISTORY OF CUPPING

While cupping therapy is most commonly associated with TCM, it has been a staple of folk medicine in many regions of the world, including Egypt, the Middle East, India, ancient Greece, and parts of Africa. It continued to be a popular treatment in Europe until the early 20th century, until it fell out of favor to conventional medicine. However, cupping is still widely used to this day in many parts of the world where conventional medicine is not as accessible.

It is thought that cupping was developed by prehistoric humans who used simple techniques, such as using the mouth to suck blood out from a wound. This was a natural instinct, just as you would suck your finger if you were pricked by a needle or a splinter. Later, instead of using their mouths, practitioners used cups. The first cups were most likely made of animal horn, which is why cupping therapy was first known as "horn therapy." To create the suction, the practitioner would suck the air out from the tip of the horn with their mouth. Some people even used the shells of pumpkins and other gourds as cups, again sucking the air from the pumpkin from a hole at the top to create suction. Later on, they used other materials, such as bamboo, clay, or earthenware cups.

One of the oldest mentions of cupping is from the Egyptian book *Ebers Papyrus*, which is the oldest medical book, written in 1550 BC. It mentions that cupping was used for treating almost every disorder, including fever, pain, vertigo, menstrual imbalances, and weakened appetite, and that it helped to accelerate healing. From Egypt, cupping was likely passed on to the ancient Greeks. Hippocrates, sometimes referred to as the father of modern medicine, used cupping for many internal and structural diseases. He was one of the first physicians to believe that disease is not due to supernatural causes, but to things of natural origin, such as poor weather, geography, poor diet, overworking, and emotions. Since the Greeks were in the Bronze Age at this time, the cups were made of bronze. At this time in history, cupping was more prominent in Greece than it was in China.

In the Middle East, many different nations use cupping for treating inflammation. Cupping is known as *hejama* or *hijama* in Arabic, which translates as "to restore to basic size" or "to diminish in volume." The founder of Islam, Muhammad, was known to be an advocate of cupping and even mentioned it throughout his writings. Muhammad wrote about cupping locations for the treatment of different pain-related diseases. Other Islamic medical texts also describe the best time to do cupping, what to eat or avoid eating before or after cupping, and how to diagnose based on cupping marks. Iranian traditional medicine uses cupping to eliminate scar tissue and holds the belief that it cleanses the internal organs.

The earliest texts of cupping in China include the following:

- The earliest record of cupping in China was found in a Han dynasty (206 BC to 220 AD) tomb, in a book called *Bo Shu*.
- The first record of cupping methods was found in a book called *Zouhou Fang*, written in 28 AD.
- The first descriptions of treatment of a specific disease were recorded in a book called *Weitaimiyao* in 755 AD, which discusses treating tuberculosis with cupping.
- Animal horns used for cupping and draining pustules from the skin were first mentioned by Ge Hong (281 to 341 AD) in *A Handbook of Prescriptions for Emergencies*.

- During the Qing dynasty (1644 to 1911 AD), Zhao Xueming wrote the *Supplement to Outline of Herbal Pharmacopoeia*, which talks about "Fire-Jar Qi," or the use of fire to create the suction for cupping, and replacing the animal horn with bamboo, ceramic, or glass cups. He also wrote about the history and origin of different kinds of cupping, different cup shapes, and their functions and applications.

In the 1950s, Chinese and Russian practitioners put a lot of research into cupping, and cupping was integrated into treatment in hospitals all over China.

Cupping was also common practice in Europe in the 19th and early 20th centuries. The Royal Marsden Hospital in London had full-time cuppers, who were often doctors or surgeons. Famous British author George Orwell wrote an essay in 1946 called "How the Poor Die," in which he describes cupping being practiced in a Parisian hospital. He writes:

> "First the doctor produced from his black bag a dozen small glasses like wine glasses, then the student burned a match inside each glass to exhaust the air, then the glass was popped on to the man's back or chest and the vacuum drew up a huge yellow blister. Only after some moments did I realize what they were doing to him. It was something called cupping, a treatment which you can read about in old medical text-books…"

By the 1880s, cupping had begun to fall out of practice in the Western world due to a lack of understanding as to how the mechanism worked, rather than the lack of therapeutic results. However, over the past few decades, cupping has shown a resurgence, and cupping therapy is practiced by a wide range of practitioners, including Traditional Chinese Medicine practitioners, acupuncturists, massage therapists, physiotherapists, chiropractors, and some medical doctors. There is no regulatory body for cupping therapy, but it may fall within the scope of practice of many different healthcare professions as an optional add-on if they get additional training.

HOW DOES CUPPING WORK?

Cupping is said to increase blood circulation, relieve pain, remove toxins from the body, and activate the immune system. So, how does it do this? The suction creates a negative pressure in the cup, which causes the soft tissue within the border of the cup to get sucked into the cup. To balance equilibrium, blood will also rush in to the area underneath the cup, which will have a lower concentration of blood than the surrounding area.

INCREASING BLOOD CIRCULATION

When blood gets sucked into the area underneath the cup, local blood circulation increases. This increased blood circulation extends down to the muscle layer, helping cells that are in the area to repair faster. This also increases granulation and angiogenesis, the formation of new connective tissue and blood vessels, during wound recovery. This can help heal soft tissue injury, relieve muscle tension, and stop pain. Cupping can draw so much blood to the area, in fact, that it can cause the capillaries in the area to severely dilate and eventually rupture, resulting in the distinctive bruising marks. The rupture of the capillaries causes bleeding, and therefore, makes it similar to autohemotherapy, which is a therapy where your own blood is drawn and re-injected into the body. It is believed to simulate the immune system, fight disease, and have healing properties.

RELIEVING PAIN

Cupping is well-known for helping to relieve pain. This could be because cupping can increase the pain threshold in the area. Another theory as to why cupping can reduce pain is the counter-irritation theory, which holds that discomfort and pain from the cupping site reduces the pain from original site. Cupping has also been shown to activate acupuncture points, and acupuncture is well-known in helping to relieve pain in a few different ways. First, it can activate small diameter nerves in the muscles, which send impulses to the spinal cord, where neurotransmitters are released to block the pain messages from reaching brain. Acupuncture can also activate the release of morphine-like endorphins, serotonin, and cortisol, which can all help to relive pain.

Cupping, much like acupuncture, can also stimulate specific nerve fibers, such as mechanosensitive A-beta fibers, which reduce pain input, and C and A-delta fibers, which inhibit pain. Cupping can also relieve pain by loosening adhesions in the muscles or fascia, the connective tissue between the skin and the muscles. Cupping lifts the fascia from the muscle, which can help reduce muscle tightness and relax the muscles. Another way cupping helps relieve pain is by bringing blood to stagnant skin and muscles, at the same time draining waste such as lactic acid from the muscles. A buildup of lactic acid can cause muscle pain and aches.

REMOVING TOXINS

Cupping has been shown to remove impure blood from the affected area. The impure blood can contain inflammatory chemicals, broken-down cells, clotted blood, scar tissue, or other substances that can cause pain and prevent healing. The increase in blood circulation in the area allows the toxins trapped in the soft tissue layers to rise to the body surface, right underneath the skin. White blood cells tend to congregate and patrol the body surface so when the toxins rise to the surface, they can quickly mop up the toxins.

Cupping has been shown to improve the immune system, as well, by causing local inflammation. Inflammatory chemicals attract white blood cells to the area and activate the complement system, a part of the immune system that enhances the ability of antibodies and white blood cells to kill off microbes and damaged cells. Cupping can also increase the level of tumor necrosis factor (TNF) and interferon, which are signaling proteins to help combat pathogens and abnormal cells in the body.

Finally, cupping can increase lymph flow. The lymphatic system is part of the immune system that helps the body get rid of toxins, waste, and other unwanted materials, and helps to circulate white blood cells throughout the body.

CUPPING, TRADITIONAL CHINESE MEDICINE, AND MODERN APPLICATIONS

According to TCM, cupping is said to improve *Qi* and Blood flow. *Qi* or *Chi* in Chinese literally means "breath," "air," or "gas." However, it can also mean "energy" or "life force." In Chinese philosophy, Qi makes up everything in the universe, both material and immaterial things. When Qi gathers together, it forms matter. Similarly, modern physics and the theory of relativity rely on Einstein's famous equation $E = mc^2$, which states that matter is made up of energy.

In the human body, Qi is needed for all metabolic functions. In modern medicine, adenosine triphosphate (ATP) is the molecule responsible for providing the energy for all metabolic functions in the body. In TCM, if Qi and Blood are unobstructed and allowed to flow freely, then there will be no disease or pain. However, if Qi and Blood flow are slowed or obstructed, this creates disease, most notably pain.

According to modern medicine, the effects of blocked Qi and Blood are analogous to what happens when someone injures themselves. Oftentimes, injuries cause bleeding. To stop the bleeding, we have platelets and blood-clotting factors that make the blood clot, preventing further bleeding and patching up the injury by making scar tissue. This blood clot and scar tissue prevent blood movement and often cause pain. Cupping is very good for treating pain because it is able to move Qi and Blood. The suction draws Qi and Blood from the surrounding areas to the affected area, and if Moving Cupping (page 22), a technique of moving the cup around the area, is used, it can move more Qi and Blood, and in larger areas.

In TCM, cupping is said to be able to remove pathogenic factors. There are six external pathogens in TCM: Wind, Cold, Heat, Dampness, Dryness, and Summer-Heat. These pathogens invade the body from the outside environment. The primary pathogen is Wind, because it can penetrate the pores of the skin and bring all the other pathogens into the body. When the pathogens attack, they produce symptoms that are similar to viral or bacterial infections in modern medicine.

We can use cupping to suck the Wind out of the body through the skin and pores, and to draw out the other pathogens along with it. The suction created by cupping can draw the lymphatic fluids, fresh blood, and white blood cells to the area, which can help kill off the virus or bacteria. Moving Cupping can stimulate the lymphatic system by pushing the lymphatic fluid through the lymph, flushing the virus or bacteria out of the body.

The external pathogens can also be caused by the weather, climate, and geographical locations we live in. One common example is damp weather causing joint pain in people with arthritis. In cold weather, muscles seize and cramp up, resulting in pain. Cupping can help remove the Dampness or Cold pathogens to help relieve pain.

Cupping is said to bring Defensive Qi to the affected area. Defensive Qi is a special type of Qi in the body that defends it against pathogens. It is similar to white blood cells in modern medicine. Defensive Qi stays near the skin surface to protect the body against the pathogens that try to invade from the outside. In modern medicine, is has been found that white blood cells often circulate just underneath the skin to patrol for invading viruses and bacteria. So, by sucking the pathogens up toward the skin, cupping draws the virus or bacteria to where the white blood cells are, waiting to attack. White blood cells are also responsible for breaking down scar tissue or adhesions that often result after an injury and cause pain.

Cupping can also help regulate organ function. If an organ is weak, gentle cupping around the organ area can help bring fresh blood supply, and with it, nutrients to nourish the organ, helping it perform more optimally. Sometimes, the internal organ function may be hindered by pathogens attacking the organ. Cupping can remove pathogens from the body to help restore the organ's function.

CHAPTER 2

CUPPING SETS

Many different types of cups can be found on the market. Each has its own unique materials, techniques for use, applications, and pros and cons. In this section, I will introduce cup types as well as how to use them, when to use them, and their pros and cons.

PLASTIC VACUUM CUPS

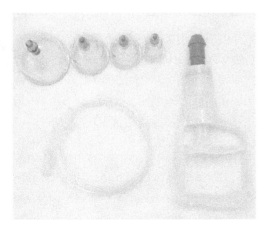

Plastic vacuum cups are clear plastic with a valve at the top. The cups usually come with rubber tubing and a hand pump. To use, attach one end of the rubber tubing to the top of the cup where the valve is, and the other end to the hand pump. Then, pull on the hand pump to suck the air out of the cups. The more pumps you apply, the more suction you will create. Generally, half a pump creates a light suction, one pump creates a medium suction, and two pumps create a strong suction.

The hand pump makes this type of cup the easiest to control, as you can control the amount of suction easily. The long rubber tubing allows you to use the cups on yourself, even on hard-to-reach places. Plastic vacuum cups are pretty versatile and can be used for all

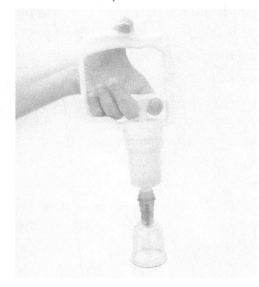

techniques, except for Moving Cupping and, in some instances, Bleeding Cupping (see page 23 for more on these techniques). The cups cannot be used for the Moving Cupping technique since the plastic rim around the cup is very sharp, which makes it hard to slide over the skin without causing pain. They cannot be used for Bleeding Cupping because blood may get into the valve at the top of the plastic cup, which cannot be disinfected properly. However, if the cups are reserved for personal use or each person has their own cups, it is okay to use them for Bleeding Cupping. To clean the cups, use warm soapy water and soak in a diluted bleach solution.

MAGNETIC CUPS

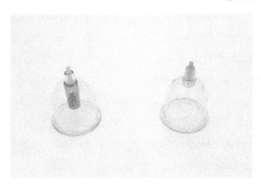

Magnetic cups are a type of plastic vacuum cup with a magnetic tip down the center. In many sets, the magnet, can be added or removed from the cups. Magnetic cups are primarily used on top of acupuncture points, as the magnet activates the acupuncture point. They are used exactly like the plastic vacuum cups, meaning they also have rubber tubing and a hand pump. The metal tips prevent the magnetic cups from sliding across the skin, as the metal tip may scratch the skin, so they cannot be used for the Moving Cupping technique. The cups are meant to stay on the skin to activate the acupuncture point, so they are not used for Flash Cupping (page 23). Magnetic cups are not generally used for Bleeding Cupping, as this would require washing the magnets regularly. They are also not used for Needle Cupping (page 25) or Moxibustion Cupping (page 26), as the magnetic tip obstructs the needle or moxibustion. To clean the cups, use warm soapy water and soak in a diluted bleach solution.

TWIST ROTARY CUPS

Twist rotary cups are another type of plastic vacuum cup but these do not require a valve or hand pump. Instead, they have a twisting rotor that expands the space in the cup, drawing the skin upward. To use, make sure the rotor is at the lowest position, then place the cup against the skin and twist the rotor upward, creating suction and drawing the skin into the cup. This cup is easy to use and to adjust the amount of suction by twisting the appropriate amount. If using for self-application, however, they are not as good as the plastic vacuum cups (page 14) or the silicone cups (below) as they may need two hands to operate (it may be hard to twist the rotor with just one hand). These cups cannot be used for Flash Cupping (page 23), because it would take too long to apply the cups. They cannot be used for Bleeding Cupping, as the twist rotary cups are hard to wash, especially if the blood gets into the rotor area. They cannot be used for Needle Cupping or Moxibustion Cupping, as the rotor would obstruct the needle and moxibustion. The moxibustion may also burn the rotor. To clean the cups, use warm soapy water, and soak in a diluted bleach solution.

SILICONE CUPS

Made of an opaque silicone material, these cups are very flexible and can be bent and compressed with ease. To use, depress the cup by pushing it downward against the skin, ejecting the air from the cup. When you let go, this will create a suction. You can easily control the amount of suction by adjusting the amount you press down. (The more you press down, the stronger the suction will be.) However, the suction on the silicone cups is not as strong as with other types. Silicone cups are great for self-application, but for people with less flexibility, they are slightly harder to manipulate than the plastic vacuum cups on areas like the back. The silicone cups are not suitable for Bleeding Cupping, as you need to use alcohol to disinfect them, but alcohol can damage the silicone material. Warm, soapy water can be used to clean the cups, but this cleaning method is not sufficient for disinfecting. Silicone cups also cannot be used for Needle Cupping or Moxibustion Cupping, as you have to press down in order to produce the suction, which will obstruct the needles or moxibustion.

GLASS CUPS

CAUTION: Do not use unless properly trained.

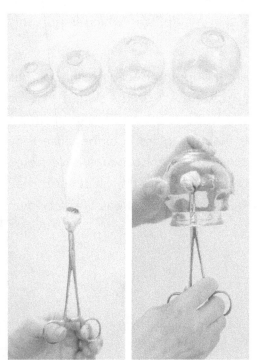

Glass cups are what most people picture when they think of cupping. These are the most widely used by TCM practitioners, although plastic cups are becoming more popular. To use, first soak a cotton ball with 95 or 99 percent alcohol. Then, hold the alcohol-soaked cotton ball with a forceps and light it on fire with a lighter or match. Stick the lit cotton ball into the glass cup for around half a second then take it out, and quickly place the cup on the affected area. The cup has to be transferred quickly or else air will go back into the cup, losing the vacuum. This technique takes training and practice, and can be dangerous if not done properly, as there is fire involved, so only qualified practitioners should use this method. The longer you leave the fire in the cup, the stronger the suction. Suction can also be controlled by using less concentrated alcohol, such as 70 percent alcohol, which will cause the fire to be weaker and create less suction. Glass cups provide the best suction out of all cups, which also makes them the most dangerous. If the suction is too strong, it may cause blistering of the skin. Glass cups are also the most versatile cups—you can apply all the techniques except Herbal Cupping using them. They are also the easiest to clean thoroughly and can be disinfected using alcohol, bleach, boiling water, or in an autoclave.

BAMBOO CUPS

CAUTION: Do not use unless properly trained.

Made of bamboo, these cups are more traditional and are rarely used today in North America. However, some specialized practitioners may still use them. Just like glass cups, suction is created in bamboo cups by soaking a cotton ball in alcohol and lighting it on fire inside of the cup. A more traditional method to create suction is lighting a piece of paper on fire, putting the paper into the cup, and then placing the cup on the skin. This method is more dangerous and very rarely used, as the fire can burn the recipient. The bamboo cups are the most difficult to use because they are not transparent, so you cannot see how much suction you have created. This is problematic and potentially damaging because if you create too much suction and leave the cups on for too long, the skin may blister, which is not only painful, but may leave scarring and lead to infection.

Bamboo cups are the only cups that can be used for Herbal Cupping because bamboo has tiny holes where it can absorb the herbs, and when the cups are left on the skin, the herbs can diffuse from the cup, into the skin, and into the body. These cups also create a strong suction, just like the glass cups. They are less versatile than the glass cups because they cannot be used for the Bleeding Cupping technique, since the bamboo cups have pores where the blood can enter, and cannot be disinfected properly. As with the glass cups, they are difficult to use for self-application, except on some easily accessible areas of the body.

CHAPTER 3

CUPPING TECHNIQUES

There are many different cupping techniques, each with its own applications and purpose. Some types of cups are suitable for some techniques but not for others.

WEAK CUPPING

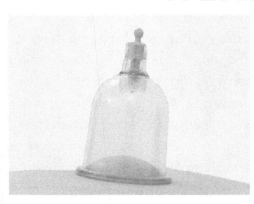

Weak Cupping can be done with any type of cup. The suction is very mild, to the point where the skin is barely sucked into the cup. There will be a mild pink color to the skin after the application. The cup should not leave any strong bruise marks, or any marks at all. If marks are left, they will fade within minutes or hours, or, at most, may take up to a couple days. This technique nourishes the body if it is depleted. It is not meant to get rid of toxins or scar tissue. It can also improve weak organ function by bringing more nutrients and blood flow to the organ to help it perform better.

This technique is good for children, the elderly, and people who are weak or have a prolonged illness. Strong suction tends to drain the body, which expends energy and resources to recover from the cupping, but Weak Cupping tends to stimulate the body, helping to regulate the blood and energy, and bring nourishment to the affected area.

When using plastic vacuum cups and magnetic cups, just pump once; even half a pump will do, as long as the cups stay on the body. For twist rotary cups, twist until the cup has a slight suction, enough to grasp onto the body. For silicone cups, press down slightly, enough to create suction with the skin. For glass cups and bamboo cups, only place the fire in the cup for half a second before placing the cup on the body. Lower concentrations of alcohol can be used to create a weaker suction. Also, the cup can be transferred slowly from the fire to the skin, which allows more air to enter the cup. For any cup type, if the suction is too strong, you can slowly lift one edge of the cup up while using one finger to lightly press down the skin, releasing some air back into the cup and reducing suction. Leave the cup on the skin for 20 to 30 minutes, checking the cups every 10 minutes to avoid blistering.

MEDIUM CUPPING

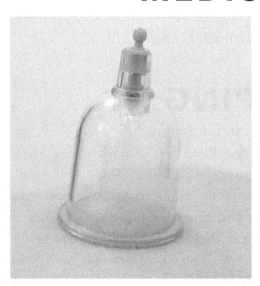

Medium Cupping is a stronger version of Weak Cupping, and a weaker version of Strong Cupping. Since it is stronger than Weak Cupping, the skin will go deeper into the cup, creating darker marks that can be dark red or even light purple in color. It is the most commonly used method of cupping, as it is good for almost all conditions. It can be used for clearing out pathogens, stopping pain, nourishing the body, and improving organ function. It can still be done on someone with a weak constitution if fewer cups are used, or if the cups are left on for less time, making it less draining on the body. It is better for pain relief compared to Weak Cupping, as stronger suction is used. It is less intense than Strong Cupping, and therefore safer. It is generally not used on the face, as it may leave bruise marks.

When using plastic vacuum cups and magnetic cups, use one full pump to create a medium amount of suction. For twist rotary cups, twist until the cup has a moderate amount of suction, enough roughly three to four twists of the rotor. For silicone cups, press down about halfway to create medium suction. For glass cups and bamboo cups, only place the fire in the cup for one second before placing it on the body. 95 to 99 percent alcohol can be used to create a medium suction. For any cup type, if the suction is too strong, you can slowly lift one edge of the cup up while using one finger to lightly press down the skin, releasing some air back into the cup and reducing suction. Leave the cups on for around 15 to 20 minutes, checking the cups every 10 minutes to avoid blistering the skin.

STRONG CUPPING

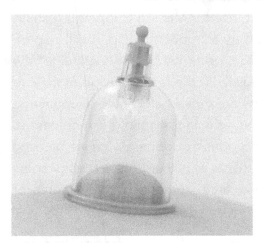

Strong Cupping can be done with any type of cup. When using, the skin is sucked deep into the cup, instantly turning it quite red. The cup may leave deep red or deep purple bruise marks, which may take a few days to a few weeks to dissipate. This technique is meant for getting rid of toxins or scar tissue. It is rather draining on the body, which will need time to repair itself and to get rid of the toxins accumulated there. This technique is good for sudden (acute) pain or injuries, sharp pain that occurs over a smaller area, and medium to strong pain. It is inappropriate to use this technique for children, the elderly, or people who are weak or have prolonged illness, as it is too draining and will tax their body.

When using plastic vacuum cups and magnetic cups, pump the cup two to three times, ensuring the skin gets sucked into the cup about an inch. For twist rotary cups, twist until the skin is sucked into the cup about an inch (three to five 180-degree twists). For silicone cups, press down all the way, so that when you let go, it creates a strong suction with the skin. For glass cups and bamboo cups, place the fire in the cup for around 1 second. You must transfer the cup quickly from the fire to the skin to ensure that a minimal amount of air goes into the cup, maintaining a strong suction. For any cup type, if the suction is not strong enough, you can take the cup off and redo it. Leave the cup on for 10 to 15 minutes.

CAUTION: If your suction is too strong, it can make the skin blister. If you feel the suction is too strong when applying the cup, slowly lift one edge of the cup up while using one finger to lightly press down on the skin, releasing some air back into the cup to reduce the suction. You must watch the skin for the duration of the session to ensure that it does not turn very dark purple or blister. If it does blister, take the cup off immediately, wash your hands with soap and warm water, and follow the instructions on page 29 under Side Effects.

MOVING CUPPING

Moving Cupping is done by sliding the cup once it has been suctioned onto the body. Use one cup at a time, and apply oil to the area before applying the cup to make it easier for it to move along the skin. Use Moving Cupping either by itself or in conjunction with Weak, Medium, or Strong Cupping. The best suction to use for Moving Cupping is usually a medium suction. If the suction is too weak, when you try to move the cup, it will pop off easily. If the suction is too strong, the cup will not budge, or it may be very painful for the person receiving the cupping. To move the cup more easily, lift the leading edge of the cup up, but not so much that air can go into the cup. Cups are moved along the acupuncture channels, or along muscles. Try not to go over bony areas, as it can be painful or unpleasant, and it is easier for the cup to pop off. Moving Cupping does not generally cause bruising marks, but is more likely to cause ecchymosis, which consists of red or purple dots or spots that appear under the skin. Move the cup along the same area for around 2 to 3 minutes, or until the area is saturated with ecchymosis.

Moving cupping is especially good for pain because it helps to release the fascia. The fascia can tighten up, causing muscle tightness and pain, or adhesions or knots, which also cause pain. Moving Cupping is very good for moving Qi and Blood. Pressing down on the cup as you move it to massage the area at the same time will also help move the Qi and Blood better, and feels similar to a massage. The speed at which you move the cup is based on a person's condition. If the person is strong or in acute pain, a faster speed and stronger pressure can be used to disperse the pain more. If the pain is not that severe, just a dull or mild ache, then lower speeds and less pressure can be used. Do not use strong Moving Cupping on people in a weak condition, as Moving Cupping tends to use up too much Qi and Blood, and can be draining on the body. However, mild Moving Cupping can help nourish the body and stimulate organ function, which can help those who are weak.

Moving Cupping can be done with nearly every cup type but is easiest with glass or silicone. The plastic cups have sharper edges, making it harder for the cups to move.

FLASH CUPPING

Flash cupping can be done with plastic cups, silicon cups, glass cups, and bamboo cups. Special training is needed if you are using glass cups or bamboo cups. If you are using glass cups, the cup will start to heat up over time. It's typically done repeatedly for 2 to 5 minutes for each area. Since the cups are removed immediately, it does not cause a lot of bruising. Generally, the area will just become red and may get some ecchymosis. This technique is used to remove toxins from the body, as well as to stop pain. Flash Cupping is good for any type of pain, especially that caused by cold or damp weather, or any changes in the weather; it's also good for colds or other infections, as it sucks the pathogen up and out of the pores.

This technique also increases blood circulation, which can help with healing, bringing nutrients to the muscles, and removing waste. It moves Qi and Blood into the area, relieving pain due to stuck Qi and Blood. Mild Flash Cupping can also be used to nourish the body, as it can bring fresh blood and nutrients to the organs, helping them to perform more optimally.

If you are cupping using a lit cotton ball, the cup will start to heat up over time. Switch to a new cup if it starts to get too warm to prevent burning the recipient. Also, the warmer the cup is, the less suction it will create.

BLEEDING CUPPING

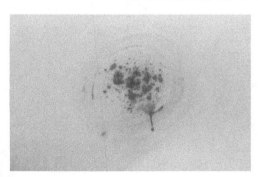

Aptly named, Bleeding Cupping draws blood out of the affected area. To do this, swab the area with 70 percent alcohol, allow it to dry, pierce the skin a few times with a lancet, then place the cup on top of the area. The vacuum will cause blood to come out of the perforated skin. Leave the cup on for around 10 minutes. Before removing the cup, wear latex or nitrile gloves to protect yourself from blood-borne pathogens. Also, have some cotton balls or gauze ready to press against the cup as you lift it, because blood may spray out if you do not cover the opening. Wipe off the blood from the skin and clean the area with 70 percent alcohol. Use new sterile gauze to bandage the area.

There will not be a lot of bruising with this technique, as the blood escapes during cupping rather than pooling up under the skin. However, mild to medium red or purple bruises may still occur.

Bleeding Cupping is very good for treating pain, especially from injuries, chronic or recurring pain, or sharp pain. The bleeding can help remove stuck or stagnated blood, which results from the body trying to repair an injury by clotting up the area. The clotted blood eventually will disappear as the white blood cells come to break it down, but oftentimes, the clot is too big and will form adhesions in the area. These adhesions and stagnated blood cause pain. Bleeding can help remove the stagnation and bring fresh blood to the area, as well as white blood cells to help break down the adhesions.

Bleeding Cupping is also excellent for treating inflammatory pain, redness, and swelling caused by inflammatory chemicals released by cells in the body during inflammation to attract white blood cells to the area. By bleeding, you can remove the inflammatory chemicals and the heat resulting from the inflammation. Bleeding Cupping is also an excellent way to reduce a fever very quickly, as fevers are also due to inflammatory chemicals.

This technique can reduce blood pressure, and can be used to treat high blood pressure. Oftentimes, Bleeding Cupping may reduce the blood pressure by 20 to 30 points after 10 minutes, depending on how much blood was extracted. But use caution for someone with low blood pressure, as fainting is also a side effect.

There's an increased risk of infection when using Bleeding Cupping, since the skin barrier will be pierced to induce bleeding. Therefore, use extra caution to disinfect the area before and after bleeding to prevent infection, especially if you or the person you are cupping is immunocompromised, or gets sick or infections easily. Do not use this technique on someone who has a bleeding or blood-clotting disorder, or people on blood thinners or anti-coagulant medication. Bleeding can also be draining on the body, so it may not be suitable for people who have a weak constitution. Some people can also faint when they see blood, so avoid it for someone who has that condition.

Typically, only glass cups are used for Bleeding Cupping, as they are the only material that can be cleaned properly for shared use without damaging the material. To clean the cups after Bleeding Cupping, wipe the blood off the cup with gauze, tissue, or cotton balls, then rinse with hot water. Then, wipe the cup with 70 percent alcohol and wash the cup in warm soapy water. Afterward, soak the cups in a diluted bleach solution overnight, and then rinse them again. Plastic or silicone cups may get damaged by alcohol, boiling water, or bleach, so they are generally not used for Bleeding Cupping. However, if the cups are not shared with anyone else, you can use the plastic vacuum cups, twist rotary cups, or silicone cups, and you can just use warm soapy water to clean and wash. Bamboo cups are not suitable for Bleeding Cupping as they have pores that can trap blood, making them impossible to clean.

NEEDLE CUPPING

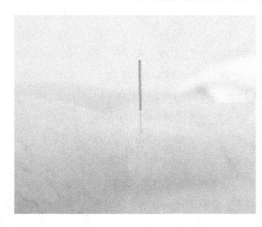

CAUTION: Do not do without proper acupuncture training.

Needle Cupping is the same as Weak or Medium Cupping, with the addition of acupuncture. To use this technique, you need knowledge of acupuncture point locations, as well as training in how to needle. Begin by inserting an acupuncture needle into an acupuncture point, then place a cup on top of the area with the needle. Generally, only weak or medium suction is used in conjunction with this technique, as strong suction may cause the needle to come out of the body. On the other hand, the opposite may happen, where strong suction may cause the handle of the needle to hit the top of the cup, making the needle go deeper into the body, which can be dangerous. Leave the cups on for around 15 to 20 minutes for the acupuncture to work. The bruise marks created will be similar to Weak Cupping or Medium Cupping.

Needle Cupping is used to improve acupuncture treatment by bringing Qi and Blood to the acupuncture point. It is useful in cases of common cold, flu, or other types of infections, as cupping can draw the pathogens to surface while the needles help the body rid itself of them. It is also used in pain management, as both acupuncture and cupping help to improve blood circulation and stop pain, therefore having a synergistic effect. Needle Cupping and acupuncture are complementary methods to improve organ function.

This technique is not used very often. Since both acupuncture and cupping are used at the same time, the chance of fainting is higher than with either method alone, so make sure the recipient has something light to eat before getting Needle Cupping done. Needle Cupping also increases the chance of the acupuncture point bleeding or bruising, as more blood is drawn to the area. If a point does bleed, just stop the bleeding with a cotton ball or cotton swab after removing the needle.

Make sure you use a taller cup that will fit on top of the needle without touching it. Magnetic cups, twist rotary cups, and silicone cups will all obstruct the needle, and therefore cannot be used for Needle Cupping.

MOXIBUSTION CUPPING

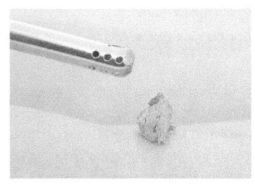

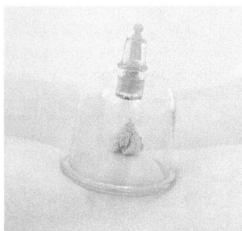

CAUTION: Do not do without proper moxibustion training.

Moxibustion Cupping is the same as Weak or Medium Cupping, with the addition of moxibustion. Moxibustion is a therapy used in TCM where a moxa made of dried mugwort (or artemisia) is burned directly, or indirectly, on the skin. You must have moxibustion training to do this method because if you are untrained, there is a high chance of burning the skin. To perform, put the moxa cone on the spot you want to cup, then light the moxa. While the moxa is lit, put a cup on top of it. Use weak or medium suction; strong cupping may cause the moxa cone to fall or tip over, which can cause a burn. A strong suction can also reduce the level of oxygen in the cup, which will extinguish the moxa. Leave the cup on for about 5 minutes, or until the area gets too hot to bear. This should only be done one cup at a time because special care needs to be used to observe how much the moxa has burned, and if the moxa gets too hot, a quick reaction time is needed to remove the cup and extinguish the moxa. Extinguish the moxa by wetting your fingers in water and pinching the moxa. If more than one moxa and cup are used at once, you may not be able to keep an eye on all of them, or determine which moxa is burning the recipient. A slow reaction to extinguish the moxa may result in a burn. If the recipient does get burned, run the burnt area under cold water, and apply some burn cream to it. Sometimes burning the skin can result in a blister. See Side Effects (page 29) for instructions on treating blisters.

Moxa is used in TCM for the treatment of most types of pain. The mugwort herb is said to be very good at moving Qi and Blood, and for relieving pain. It is especially useful for pain that feels cold to the touch, gets worse in cold weather, or feels better with warmth, since moxa is warm when it burns. In addition to helping move Qi and Blood, this warming effect also dilates the blood vessels in the area, increasing blood circulation. Moxa is also good for getting rid of certain types of acute infections, especially the type where you feel chills. It can nourish the body and help improve organ function. In fact, it is the primary method of tonifying the body in acupuncture. Therefore, it is suitable for people with weak constitutions.

Glass cups are best to use, as glass will not burn and you can visually observe how much of the moxa has burned and avoid burning the skin. Bamboo can be used, but it is not see-through so there is a higher chance of burns. Though transparent, plastic cups may melt if the moxa is too close to it. You may be able to use plastic for Moxibustion Cupping if you use a larger cup. Silicone cups, magnetic cups, and twist rotary cups will all obstruct the moxa cone, and therefore are not suitable for Moxibustion Cupping.

HERBAL CUPPING

CAUTION: Do not use unless you have herbal training and training with bamboo cups.

Herbal Cupping consists of soaking bamboo cups in a hot herbal decoction before applying them to the skin. The pores inside the bamboo cups will absorb the herbal decoction, and the skin will absorb the active ingredients as the cup stays on the body. Herbal decoctions will vary depending on the recipient's condition. If the recipient has pain, herbs that relieve pain are used. If the recipient has an infection, herbs that kill pathogens are used. If the recipient is weak and needs nourishing, herbs that improve organ function are used. The herbs will enhance the effects of the cupping. Weak, medium, or strong suction can be used based on the recipient's condition. The cups are retained for around 20 minutes in order for the body to absorb the herbs. The bruise marks made by the cups will depend on the amount of suction used. Proper training with bamboo cups is a must, as bamboo cups are the hardest to use and may cause the most side effects if suction is too strong.

WATER CUPPING

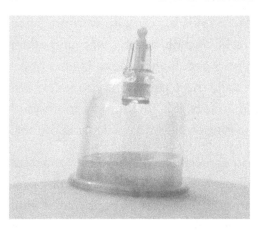

Water Cupping consists of adding an ounce of water to the cups before applying them to the body. The cups have to be applied quickly to avoid spilling the water, which may take some practice. Weak, medium, or strong suction is then applied to the cups. Leave on for 15 to 20 minutes before removing. When removing, be sure to have a dry towel ready, as the water will spill out once the cups are removed. It's best to lift only one side of the cup, and then press the towel against the same side so that the towel will catch all the water. Bruise marks from Water Cupping are generally mild, and usually just some redness will occur.

An excellent way to cool the body down very quickly, Water Cupping is good for pain that feels better with cold, such as inflammatory pain that is red, swollen, and feels hot to the touch. It's also good at reducing a fever quickly, as the water will cool the body down. It can also be used to cool down someone who has a lot of heat in the body. Signs of this include always feeling hot, having a tendency to drink cold water, and producing a lot of smelly or oily sweat. Do not use on people who have a colder constitution, as it may make them colder. Water Cupping is also used for those who are very dry, with symptoms such as dry skin, dry throat, dry hair, and constipation. The water can be absorbed through the skin to help supplement the lack of water in the body.

CHAPTER 4

SAFETY

Cupping is generally very safe, and the chance of side effects is rare. According to a systematic review of 550 clinical studies about cupping, published in the *Journal of Traditional Chinese Medical Sciences*, an adverse reaction was reported in only one incident. However, the clinical studies were done by trained professionals. Nevertheless, with the exception of using glass or bamboo cups and some of the more specialized techniques described in the previous chapter, cupping is pretty easy to do, even for people who are not trained. Many cultures use it as a home remedy, passed on from generation to generation. With the inventions of the new plastic and silicone cups that are very easy to use, cupping is accessible to everyone.

SIDE EFFECTS

The most common side effect is the bruising marks made by the cups. However, this is a desired effect of cupping, as it indicates that the toxins are getting drawn out, and is not really considered a side effect. The bruise marks can become red or even purple, which is still okay, as long as the bruise is not deep purple or black, which may indicate the cup was left on for too long or the suction was too strong. To prevent this, never leave the cups on for longer than 20 minutes, and check on them every 5 minutes in case the cups need to be removed early due to intense bruising. Much like a regular bruise, bruising from cupping can feel sore or tender, which is normal.

If cups are left on for too long or if the suction is too strong, blisters can form. If you see a blister forming, remove the cups immediately. If the blister is large, disinfect the blister and the surrounding area with 70 percent alcohol. Sterilize a sewing needle with 70 percent alcohol, boiling water, or a lighter, and use it to poke a couple of holes in the blister. Use a sterile gauze pad, using it to press on the blister and drain it out. Disinfect the blister again, and bandage it up with a new sterile gauze pad. Seek medical attention immediately from your medical doctor. Small blisters will reabsorb into the body over time.

Cupping also comes with a risk of fainting. Cupping is relaxing and can lower the blood pressure. If the blood pressure drops too low, it can cause people to faint. Signs of fainting include nausea, cold sweat, light-headedness, dizziness, cold extremities, or feeling cold. If you feel signs of fainting during a cupping treatment, remove the cups immediately, lie down with feet elevated, cover yourself with blankets, and drink some warm or hot water. Eating or drinking something sugary, such as candy of fruit juice, can help as well. To prevent fainting, have a light snack before cupping. Do not eat too much, either. Do not do cupping when feeling tired or drained. If someone is very weak, they should not use strong cupping, as it increases the chances of fainting. If someone is very nervous about cupping, this can increase chances of fainting, so make sure you are calm and relaxed before receiving a cupping treatment.

During cupping, there should not be any pain. Sometimes pain is present if your muscles are very tight, or if you already have a lot of pain in the area. In that case, do not use strong suction. Use just enough suction to handle without causing pain. If you do feel pain from the cups, it generally means the suction is too strong, so you can lift up the side of the cup a little bit to let in some air and reduce some of the vacuum. Alternatively, you can take the cup off and redo it. An exception to this is with Moving Cupping, when some pain is to be expected. To reduce the pain, use plenty of oil on the area you want to do Moving Cupping. Also, doing it at a slower speed can reduce the pain.

CAUTIONS AND CONTRAINDICATIONS

Caution should be used for people who are weak or with a poor constitution. They are more susceptible to fainting. Less suction should be used to make sure they are not drained. When using Moving Cupping, the cups should not be moved aggressively, but in a milder or gentler way.

Caution should also be used for pregnant women. Do not do any cupping on the abdomen, the mid to lower back, or the sacrum. Some acupuncture points are also contraindicated for pregnancy. If in doubt, it is better not to do any cupping on pregnant women. Cupping should also be used with caution for a woman who is menstruating, as it may be too draining on her or may prolong her menstruation. Wait for menstruation to stop before doing cupping.

Cupping should not be done on any of the following:

- Areas where there are major arteries, or where a pulse can be felt

- Areas with edema

- Areas with skin disorders or open sores, such as sunburn, scrapes, cuts, etc.

- Joints with very little muscle covering them, like the back of the elbow or the top of the knee

- On a blood clot, such as deep vein thrombosis, as dislodging the blood clot can be dangerous

- On broken or fractured bones

- On cancer tumors, fibroids, cysts, or other nodules

- Someone who has a high fever

- Someone who is convulsing, or whose muscles are in spasm

- Someone with bleeding disorders or on blood thinners

- The nipples or any orifices of the body (e.g., eyes, mouth, anus)

If you are not trained to use fire to induce a vacuum, do not try it. If you are trained to do it, be cautious with the fire around others. Always have a fire extinguisher in the room. Do not soak your cotton ball with too much alcohol; it just has to be moist throughout. Do not wear loose clothing, as it may catch on fire. Tie up long hair so it does not catch fire. Make sure there are no other flammable objects nearby, as well. Use a bowl of water to put out the fire from the cotton ball, instead of trying to blow it out. Do not travel around with the lit cotton ball, so make sure you have everything you need close by. Do not handle the lit cotton ball over the body. If someone is burned, sterilize and bandage the area with sterile gauze and go see a doctor.

Bleeding Cupping comes with an increased risk of infection, since the skin barrier will be pierced to induce bleeding. Therefore, use extra caution to disinfect the area before and after bleeding to prevent infection. When doing Bleeding Cupping, make sure to wear gloves to protect yourself from blood-borne infections. Wipe the area clean with 70 percent alcohol, and let it dry before piercing the skin. After Bleeding Cupping, clean the area of with sterile gauze, then wipe it again with 70 percent alcohol. Bandage up the area with new sterile gauze.

CLEANING AND DISINFECTING

For cups that are not used for Bleeding Cupping or Needle Cupping and only touch intact skin (i.e., skin with no cuts or breaks), you can clean them using warm, soapy water. Since they will not be in contact with blood, the cups do not need to be disinfected.

If the cups were used after needling, or if there is some break in the skin, then they need to be disinfected. Wipe the cups off with a 70 percent alcohol solution. Wash the cups in warm, soapy water. Soak the cups in a diluted bleach solution, using 1:50 bleach-to-water solution for 20 minutes, and then rinse the cups.

If the cups were used for Bleeding Cupping, rinse the cup with hot water. Wipe the cup with 70 percent alcohol. Wash the cup in warm, soapy water. Soak the cups in a 1:50 bleach-to-water solution overnight, and then rinse the cups.

Alcohol should not be used on plastic cups or silicone cups, as it may deteriorate the material very fast, so it is best not to do Bleeding Cupping with these cups. If the cups are not shared between individuals, then they can just be cleaned with warm, soapy water.

CHAPTER 5

TREATMENT OF SPORTS INJURIES AND PAIN MANAGEMENT

Cupping is most well-known for the treatment of pain. In fact, according to the *Journal of Traditional Chinese Medical Sciences*, it has been found that cupping therapy, either alone or combined with other interventions, was better than medication or other interventions alone for treating many types of pain. The main reason it is so successful in treating pain compared to only medication is that most medications just mask the pain and do not fix the underlying issue. Cupping, however, not only can help stop the pain, but also helps your body to repair itself, addressing the underlying problem causing the pain, whether it is an injury, tightness, or adhesions, etc.

In How Does Cupping Work? (page 10), I described many reasons how cupping can relieve pain and promote healing. Cupping can also relieve muscle tension, help release the fascia, and physically break up adhesions or knots. Moving Cupping and Flash Cupping are especially good at doing this, as they help to massage the area. Images in this chapter and in Chapter 6 will have arrows to show how to use Moving Cupping, if you decide to use this technique, for the points being discussed.

Cupping not only works on the muscles, but can activate the nerves that help block pain signals, as well. It can help nerves release certain neurotransmitters and endorphins, which help to stop the sensation of pain. Cupping also increases pain threshold, which means more stimulus is needed to trigger pain.

Cupping activates acupuncture points, so they are often placed on acupuncture points to maximize their effectiveness. Of course, most people do not know where acupuncture points are located, so this book will tell you how to find them. Generally, it is best to use the hand of the person being treated instead of inches as the reference tool to find the points, since everyone is different in size. For an adult close to your height, you can use your own hand as the reference tool to simplify things. If they are taller or shorter than you are, and their hand is much bigger or smaller than your hand, then adjust your measurements as needed.

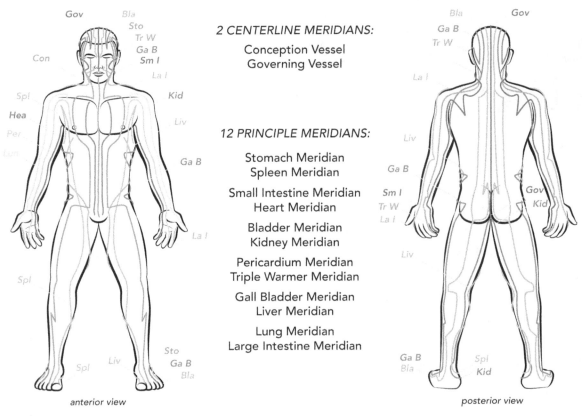

2 CENTERLINE MERIDIANS:

Conception Vessel
Governing Vessel

12 PRINCIPLE MERIDIANS:

Stomach Meridian
Spleen Meridian

Small Intestine Meridian
Heart Meridian

Bladder Meridian
Kidney Meridian

Pericardium Meridian
Triple Warmer Meridian

Gall Bladder Meridian
Liver Meridian

Lung Meridian
Large Intestine Meridian

anterior view   posterior view

Body meridians

You can also use anatomical landmarks to find the acupuncture points. I will use some anatomical terminology to locate these points in relation to anatomical landmarks. Some terms that I may use and what they mean are:

Superior: Above something or upper portion of something

Inferior: Below something or lower portion of something

Midline: Center of the body

Lateral: Away from the midline; on the outer side of the body

Medial: Toward the midline; on the inner side of the body

Posterior: Toward the back of the body

Anterior: Toward the front of the body

Distal: Away from the body or toward the extremities

Proximal: Toward the body, or away from the extremities

Some knowledge about bone names or muscle names will be very useful when finding the points, as well, particularly the vertebral column. I will use the anatomical names of the muscles and bones, as well as common known names where possible.

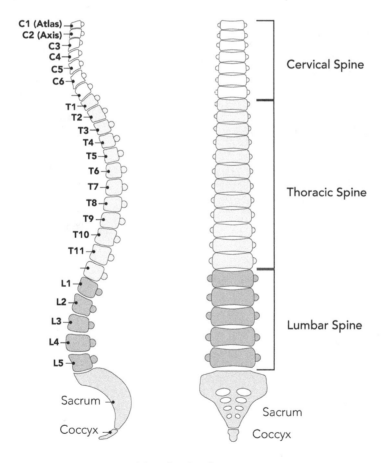

Vertebral column

In Chapter 3: Cupping Techniques, I describe different techniques that are good for different types of pain. Each topic discussed below will refer to those, so it would be helpful to familiarize yourself with the material in that chapter before continuing.

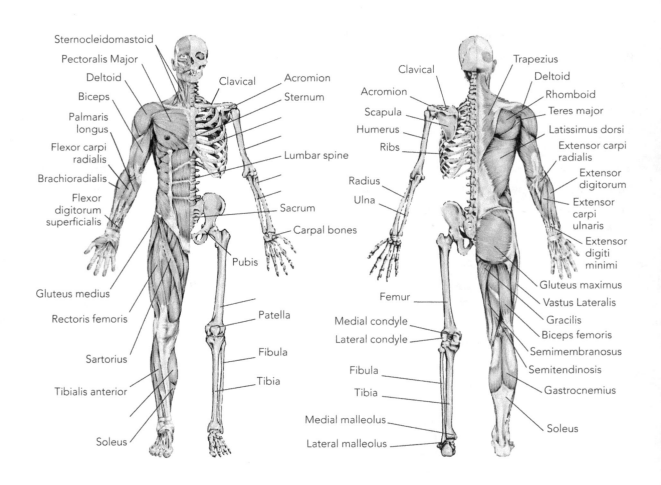

Musculoskeletal system

NECK AND SHOULDER PAIN

Neck and shoulder pain are the most common types of pain, and the cause is usually not due to injury, but to poor posture. If the posture is not fixed, neck pain will keep coming back, so make a conscious effort to notice your posture. Other causes of neck pain include whiplash (from sports injuries or car accidents), cervical degeneration, stress, and infections such as colds or flu.

In TCM, neck and shoulder pain, in addition to the causes mentioned above, is due to the obstruction of Qi and Blood movement in the meridians, which causes pain. This can be due to pathogenic Wind or Cold. Obstruction can also be due to trauma or stress.

GB20 *Feng Chi–Wind Pool*

Location: In the depression between the sternocleidomastoid muscle and the trapezius muscle, just at the base of the skull.

Affected muscles: Trapezius, semispinalis, splenius.

When to use: For any type of neck and/or shoulder pain, especially due to stress, tension, using the computer a lot, or cold or flu.

Application: GB20 is actually within the hairline, so a cup cannot be

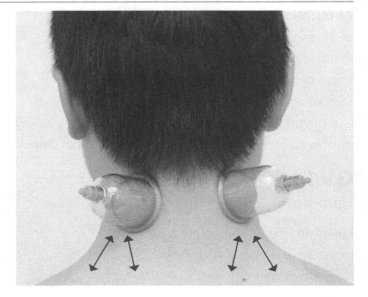

placed directly on it. Instead, place the cup as close to the hairline as possible. Apply Weak or Medium Cupping for 10 to 15 minutes. Use stronger suction for acute or severe pain, and weaker for mild or chronic pain. Use Flash Cupping if neck pain is due to a cold. Apply Moving Cupping up and down the neck from GB20 for 30 seconds per cup to effectively relieve neck tension caused by acute pain, stress, or injury.

GB21 *Jian Jing–Shoulder Well*

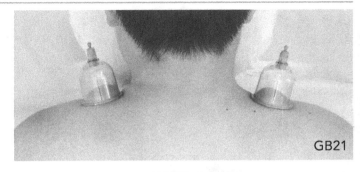
GB21

Location: On the most superior part of the shoulder, directly above the nipple, or halfway from the spine to the deltoid muscle.

Affected muscles: Trapezius.

When to use: For any type of neck and/or shoulder pain, especially due to stress, tension, using the computer a lot, or cold or flu.

Application: Apply Weak, Medium, or Strong Cupping for 10 to 15 minutes. Use stronger suction for acute or severe pain, and weaker for mild or chronic pain. Use Flash

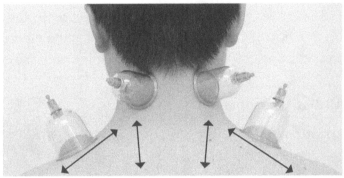

Cupping if neck pain is due to a cold. Apply Moving Cupping sideways across the trapezius muscle to loosen up the muscle, and to relieve neck and shoulder pain.

GV14 *Da Zhui–Great Hammer*

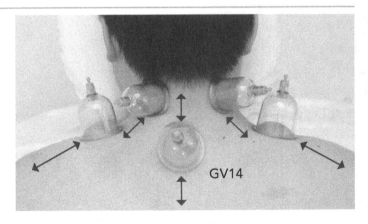
GV14

Location: Below the spinous process of the seventh cervical vertebra (C7), approximately level with the acromion (shoulders).

Affected muscles: Trapezius, rhomboid minor, serratus posterior superior.

When to use: For any type of neck and/or shoulder pain, especially due to stress, tension, using the computer a lot, or cold or flu. Also used when there is a burning pain.

Application: Apply Weak, Medium, or Strong Cupping for 10 to 15 minutes. Use stronger suction for acute or severe pain, and weaker for mild or chronic pain. Use Flash Cupping if neck pain is due to a cold. Apply Moving Cupping up and down the spine, and sideways across the trapezius, to relieve tension in the neck and shoulder. Use Bleeding Cupping on GV14 to relieve pain and inflammation quickly, especially if a burning sensation accompanies neck and shoulder pain.

BL12 *Feng Men—Wind Gate*

Location: About 1.5 inches on either side of the spinous process of the second thoracic vertebra (T2).

Affected muscles: Trapezius, rhomboid minor, rhomboid major, erector spinae, semispinalis capitis, semispinalis cervicis, serratus posterior superior.

When to use: For any type of neck and/or shoulder pain, especially due to stress, tension, using the computer a lot, or cold or flu.

Application: Apply Weak, Medium, or Strong Cupping for 10 to 15 minutes. Use stronger suction for acute or severe pain, and weaker for mild or chronic pain. Use Flash Cupping if neck pain is due to a cold. Apply Moving Cupping up and down the erector spinae to relieve shoulder and upper back pain.

BL13 *Fei Shu—Lung Shu*

Location: About 1.5 inches on either side of the spinous process of the third thoracic vertebra (T3).

Affected muscles: Trapezius, rhomboid minor, rhomboid major, erector spinae, semispinalis cervicis, semispinalis thoracis, serratus posterior superior.

When to use: For any type of neck 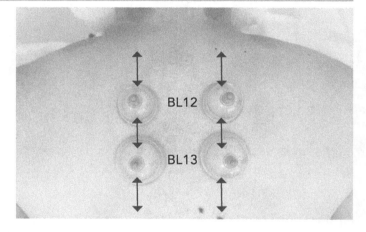 and/or shoulder pain, especially due to stress, tension, using the computer a lot, or cold or flu.

Application: Apply Weak, Medium, or Strong Cupping for 10 to 15 minutes. Use stronger suction for acute or severe pain, and weaker for mild or chronic pain. Use Flash Cupping if neck pain is due to a cold. Use Moving Cupping up and down the erector spinae to relieve shoulder and upper back pain. Use Bleeding Cupping on BL13 to relieve upper back pain quickly.

SHOULDER JOINT PAIN

A very complicated joint that connects the humerus, scapula, and clavicle, the shoulder is easily injured by frequent use. The muscles around the shoulder joint are often referred to as the rotator cuff, and they include the supraspinatus, infraspinatus, teres minor, and subscapularis. Cupping is very good for relieving inflammation from bursitis, tendonitis, dislocation, and frozen shoulder; it also is very effective at breaking down the scarring from rotator cuff injuries. You can also use cupping for those suffering from arthritis. Although arthritis is a degenerative disorder, in TCM, it is thought to be a buildup of Damp pathogen in the joints. Cupping can help remove the Damp pathogen from the joint, helping it heal.

Jianqian *Front of the Shoulder*

Location: Front of the shoulder, midway between the end of the axilla (armpit) and the lateral end of the clavicle, where the deltoid muscles attach.

Affected muscles: Deltoid, pectoralis major, coracobrachialis, latissimus dorsi, biceps brachii.

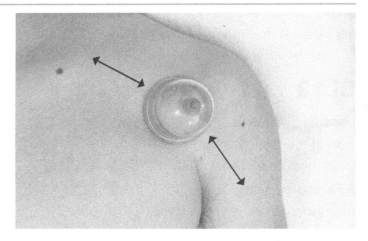

When to use: For any type of anterior shoulder joint pain, or pain in the front of the shoulder. Used often for frozen shoulder, tendonitis, or arthritis of the shoulder joint.

Application: Apply Weak, Medium, or Strong Cupping for 10 to 15 minutes. Use stronger suction for acute or severe pain, and weaker for mild or chronic pain. Apply Moving Cupping up and down the arm to increase circulation, relieve inflammation, and relieve scarring. Use Flash Cupping to help relieve pain. Use Bleeding Cupping for stubborn shoulder pain.

LI15 *Jian Yu—Shoulder Bone*

Location: Just lateral to the acromion, on the upper anterior portion of the deltoid muscle.

Affected muscles: Deltoid.

When to use: For any type of lateral shoulder pain, or pain on the sides of the shoulder. Used often for frozen shoulder, tendonitis, or strain injury of the deltoid.

Application: Apply Weak, Medium, or Strong Cupping for 10 to 15 minutes. Use stronger suction for acute or severe pain, and weaker for mild or chronic pain. Use Moving Cupping up and down the deltoid for increasing circulation, relieving inflammation, and relieving scarring.

TE14 *Jian Liao–Shoulder Bone Hole*

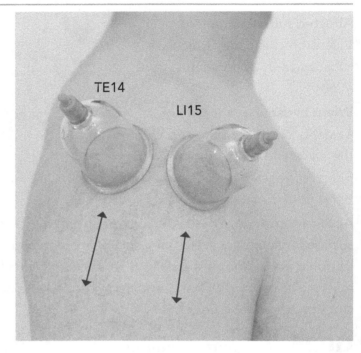

Location: Just lateral to the acromion, on the upper posterior portion of the deltoid muscle, an inch behind LI15.

Affected muscles: Deltoid.

When to use: For any type of lateral shoulder pain, or pain on the sides of the shoulder. Used often for frozen shoulder, tendonitis, or strain injury of the deltoid.

Application: Apply Weak, Medium, or Strong Cupping for 10 to 15 minutes. Use stronger suction for acute or severe pain, and weaker for mild or chronic pain. Apply Moving Cupping up and down the deltoid for increasing circulation, relieving inflammation, and relieving scarring.

SI9 *Jian Zhen–True Shoulder*

Location: On the back, 1 inch above the axillary (armpit) fold when the arm is relaxed.

Affected muscles: Deltoid, latissimus dorsi, teres major, triceps brachii, subscapularis, infraspinatus, teres minor.

When to use: For any type of posterior shoulder pain, or pain on the back of the shoulder joint. Used often for frozen shoulder, tendonitis, or rotator cuff injury.

Application: Apply Weak, Medium, or Strong Cupping for 10 to 15 minutes. Use stronger suction for acute or severe pain, and weaker for mild or chronic pain. Apply Moving Cupping up and down the deltoid for increasing circulation, relieving inflammation, and relieving scarring. Do Flash Cupping to help relieve pain.

SI10 *Nao Shu–Upper Arm Shu*

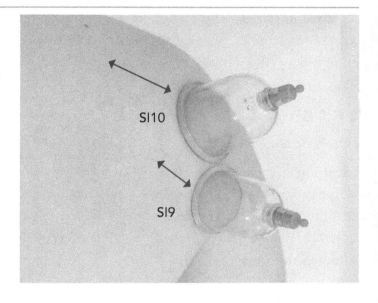

Location: On the back, 1 inch above SI9, or just below the acromion.

Affected muscles: Deltoid, triceps brachii, coracobrachialis, subscapularis, infraspinatus, teres minor.

When to use: For any type of posterior shoulder pain, or pain on the back of the shoulder joint. Used often for frozen shoulder, tendonitis, or rotator cuff injury.

Application: Apply Weak, Medium, or Strong Cupping for 10 to 15 minutes. Use stronger suction for acute or severe pain, and weaker for mild or chronic pain. Apply Moving Cupping up and down the deltoid for increasing circulation, relieving inflammation, and relieving scarring. Do Flash Cupping to help relieve pain. Use Bleeding Cupping for stubborn shoulder pain.

GB21 *Jian Jing–Shoulder Well*

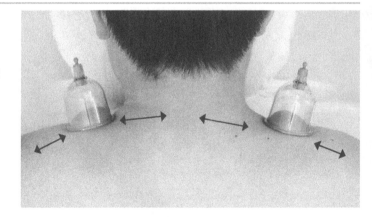

Location: On the most superior part of the shoulder, directly above the nipple, or halfway from the spine to the deltoid.

Affected muscles: Trapezius.

When to use: For any type of superior shoulder pain, or pain on the top of the shoulder joint. Used often when there is shoulder stiffness as a result of shoulder joint pain.

Application: Apply Weak, Medium, or Strong Cupping for 10 to 15 minutes. Use stronger suction for acute or severe pain, and weaker for mild or chronic pain. Use Flash Cupping if neck pain is due to a cold. Apply Moving Cupping sideways across the trapezius muscle to loosen up the muscle and relieve shoulder joint pain.

ELBOW PAIN

The two most common types of elbow pain are tennis elbow (lateral epicondylitis) and golfer's elbow (medial epicondylitis). Tennis elbow affects the lateral, or outside, part of the elbow. It is usually due to repetitive motions, incorrect movement of the arms, or damage to the muscles or tendons from carrying heavy objects. Most people who have tennis elbow are not athletes but still use their arms a lot, such as plumbers, painters, carpenters, butchers, chefs, or those whose work involves using a computer mouse. Golfer's elbow affects the medial, or inside, part of the elbow. This is not as common as tennis elbow, but the causes are the same. The motions that affect the muscles that attach to the medial epicondyle involve gripping, which can occur with golfing, throwing a ball, rock climbing, or using tools. Other causes of elbow pain can include rheumatism, rheumatoid arthritis, or trauma.

LI11 *Qu Chi–Pool at the Bend*

Location: When the elbow is half flexed, the point where the lateral elbow crease ends.

Affected muscles: Extensor carpi radialis longus, extensor carpi radialis brevis, brachialis, brachioradialis, supinator.

When to use: For any type of lateral elbow pain. Used often for tennis elbow or arthritis of the elbow.

Application: Apply Weak, Medium, or Strong Cupping for 10 to 15 minutes. Use stronger suction for acute or severe pain, and weaker for mild or chronic pain. Apply Moving Cupping up and down the forearm for tennis elbow. Do Flash Cupping to help relieve pain. Use Bleeding Cupping on the blood vessels close to LI11 to quickly relieve elbow pain.

LI10 *Shou San Li–Arm Three Mile*

Location: Three fingers' width (or two inches) below LI11.

Affected muscles: Extensor carpi radialis longus, extensor carpi radialis brevis, supinator, brachioradialis.

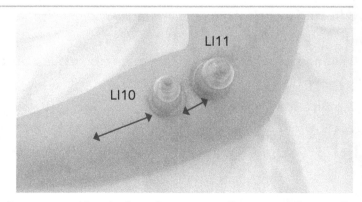

When to use: For any type of lateral elbow pain. Used often for tennis elbow or arthritis of the elbow.

Application: Apply Weak, Medium, or Strong Cupping for 10 to 15 minutes. Use stronger suction for acute or severe pain, and weaker for mild or chronic pain. Apply Moving Cupping up and down the forearm for tennis elbow.

HT3 *Shao Hai–Lesser Sea*

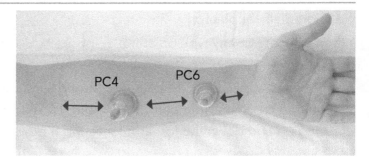

Location: When the elbow is half flexed, the point where the medial elbow crease ends.

Affected muscles: Pronator teres, brachialis.

When to use: For any type of medial elbow pain. Used often for golfer's elbow or arthritis of the elbow.

Application: Apply Weak, Medium, or Strong Cupping for 10 to 15 minutes. Use stronger suction for acute or severe pain, and weaker for mild or chronic pain. Apply Moving Cupping up and down the forearm for golfer's elbow. Use Flash Cupping to help relieve pain. Use Bleeding Cupping on the blood vessels close to HT3 to quickly relieve pain.

PC4 *Xi Men–Cleft Gate*

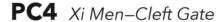

Location: About 1 inch (or one thumb's width) below the halfway point of the inner part of the forearm, in between the two tendons of the palmaris longus and flexor carpi radialis.

Affected muscles: Flexor carpi radialis, palmaris longus, flexor digitorum sublimis, flexor digitorum profundus.

When to use: For any type of medial elbow pain. Used often for golfer's elbow or arthritis of the elbow.

Application: Apply Weak, Medium, or Strong Cupping for 10 to 15 minutes. Use stronger suction for acute or severe pain, and weaker for mild or chronic pain. Apply Moving Cupping up and down the forearm for golfer's elbow.

FOREARM OR WRIST PAIN

The most common cause of forearm pain is wrist or elbow pain or injuries. Carpal tunnel syndrome is due to the compression of the median nerve, which causes pain, numbness, and a tingling sensation in the fingers. The incidence of carpal tunnel is increasing because of the prevalent use of computer keyboards and mice. Brachial plexus injury, which is actually an injury to the neck that in turn injures the nerves that control the arm, can cause arm pain. A major cause of brachial plexus injury is whiplash from car accidents or sports injuries. For treating neck pain, see Neck and Shoulder Pain (page 37).

LI11 *Qu Chi—Pool at the Bend*

Location: When the elbow is half flexed, the point where the elbow crease ends on the outside of the elbow.

Affected muscles: Extensor carpi radialis longus, extensor carpi radialis brevis, brachialis, brachioradialis, supinator.

When to use: For any type of lateral forearm pain. Used often for carpal tunnel syndrome, or when using the computer mouse or typing too much, or people who use their hands to grip tools a lot.

Application: Apply Weak, Medium, or Strong Cupping for 10 to 15 minutes. Use stronger suction for acute or severe pain, and weaker for mild or chronic pain. Use Moving Cupping up and down the forearm for forearm pain. Use Flash cupping to help relieve pain. Use Bleeding Cupping on the blood vessels close to LI11 to quickly relieve pain.

LI10 *Shou San Li—Arm Three Mile*

Location: Three fingers' width (or 2 inches) below LI11.

Affected muscles: Extensor carpi radialis longus, extensor carpi radialis brevis, supinator, brachioradialis.

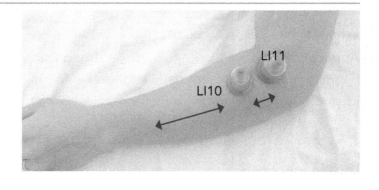

When to use: For any type of lateral forearm pain. Used often for carpal tunnel syndrome, or when using the computer mouse or typing too much, or people who use their hands to grip tools a lot.

Application: Apply Weak, Medium, or Strong Cupping for 10 to 15 minutes. Use stronger suction for acute or severe pain, and weaker for mild or chronic pain. Use Moving Cupping up and down the forearm for forearm pain.

TE5 *Wai Guan—Outer Pass*

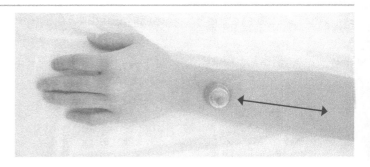

Location: The lateral part of the forearm, about three fingers' width (or 2 inches) above the wrist crease, between the radius and ulna bones.

Affected muscles: Extensor indicis, extensor pollicis longus, extensor pollicis brevis, extensor carpi ulnaris, extensor digiti minimi, extensor digitorum.

When to use: For any type of medial forearm pain. Used often for carpal tunnel syndrome.

Application: Apply Weak or Medium Cupping for 10 to 15 minutes. Use stronger suction for acute or severe pain, and weaker for mild or chronic pain. Use Moving Cupping up and down the forearm for forearm pain and carpal tunnel syndrome.

HT3 *Shou Hai—Lesser Sea*

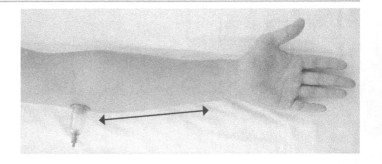

Location: When the elbow is half flexed, the point where the medial elbow crease ends. Treat while arm is straight.

Affected muscles: Pronator teres, brachialis.

When to use: For any type of medial forearm pain.

Application: Apply Weak, Medium, or Strong Cupping for 10 to 15 minutes. Use stronger suction for acute or severe pain, and weaker for mild or chronic pain. Use Moving Cupping up and down the forearm for forearm pain. Do Flash Cupping to help relieve pain.

PC4 *Xi Men—Cleft Gate*

Location: About one thumb's width (or 1 inch) below the halfway point of the inner part of the forearm, in between the two tendons of the palmaris longus and flexor carpi radialis.

Affected muscles: Flexor carpi radialis, palmaris longus, flexor digitorum sublimis, flexor digitorum profundus.

When to use: For any type of medial forearm pain. Used often for carpal tunnel syndrome.

Application: Apply Weak, Medium, or Strong Cupping for 10 to 15 minutes. Use stronger suction for acute or severe pain, and weaker for mild or chronic pain. Use Moving Cupping up and down the forearm for forearm pain and carpal tunnel syndrome.

PC6 *Nei Guan—Inner Pass*

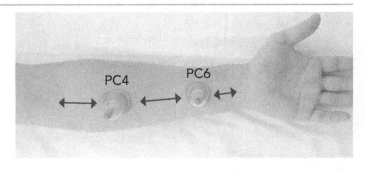

Location: The inside part of the forearm, about 2 inches (or 3 fingers' width) above the wrist crease between the two prominent tendons (palmaris longus and flexor carpi radialis).

Affected muscles: Brachioradialis, flexor digitorum profundus, flexor digitorum superficialis, flexor carpi radialis, palmaris longus.

When to use: For any type of medial forearm pain. Used often for carpal tunnel syndrome.

Application: Apply Weak or Medium Cupping for 10 to 15 minutes. Use stronger suction for acute or severe pain, and weaker for mild or chronic pain. Use Moving Cupping up and down the forearm for carpal tunnel syndrome.

CHEST PAIN

Heart, lung, gastrointestinal, and musculoskeletal problems can all cause chest pain. In this section, I will focus on musculoskeletal chest pain, which is mainly due to damage or injury to the pectoralis major muscle, often from weight lifting with poor posture or while using heavy weights. Soft tissue injury or bruised or broken ribs from accidents or falls can also cause chest pain. A rib injury will feel worse with deep breathing or coughing, is very localized to one area/rib, and feels sore when pressed.

Chest pain that cannot be explained by injury may be due to something else, such as a heart or lung problem. These can be serious and even life-threatening, so it is always a good idea to see your medical doctor for an unexplainable chest pain.

LU2 *Yun Men—Pool at the Bend*

Location: On the lateral side of the chest, below the clavicle, just under the deltopectoral triangle. The deltopectoral triangle is an indentation formed by the deltoid, pectoral muscle, and clavicle; it can be found if you raise your arm forward and upward 90 degrees.

Affected muscles: Deltoid, pectoralis major.

When to use: For chest pain or pain of the pectoral muscle. Especially useful for chest pain due to respiratory issues.

Application: Apply Weak, Medium, or Strong Cupping for 10 to 15 minutes. Use stronger suction for acute or severe pain, and weaker for mild or chronic pain. Apply Moving Cupping across the chest for chest pain. Use Flash Cupping to help relieve pain.

LU1 *Zhong Fu—Central Palace*

Location: About 1 inch below LU2.

Affected muscles: Deltoid, pectoralis major.

When to use: For chest pain or pain of the pectoral muscle. Especially useful for chest pain due to respiratory issues.

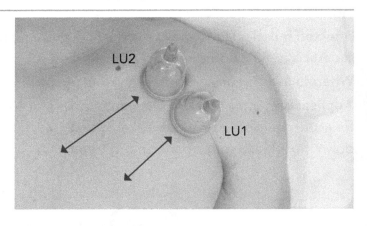

Application: Apply Weak, Medium, or Strong Cupping for 10 to 15 minutes. Use stronger suction for acute or severe pain, and weaker for mild or chronic pain. Apply Moving Cupping across the chest for chest pain. Use Flash Cupping to help relieve pain.

ST15 *Wu Yi—Roof*

Location: In the second intercostal space, approximately above the nipples.

Affected muscles: Pectoralis major.

When to use: For chest pain or pain of the pectoral muscle, or pain in the intercostals. Especially useful for

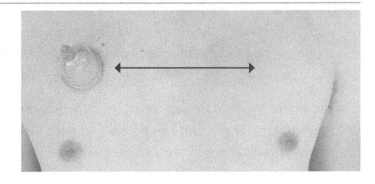

chest pain due to respiratory issues, as well as for breast pain.

Application: Apply Weak, Medium, or Strong Cupping for 10 to 15 minutes. Use stronger suction for acute or severe pain, and weaker for mild or chronic pain. Use Moving Cupping across the chest for chest pain. Use Flash Cupping to help relieve pain.

SP21 *Da Bao–Great Embracement*

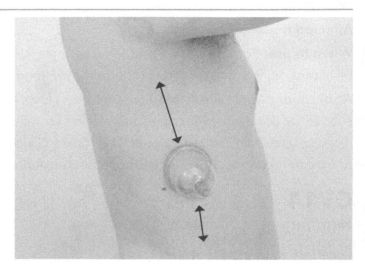

Location: On the side of the chest, midway between the axilla (armpit) and the twelfth rib.

Affected muscles: Latissimus dorsi, serratus anterior.

When to use: For pain on the side of the chest.

Application: Apply Weak, Medium, or Strong Cupping for 10 to 15 minutes. Use stronger suction for acute or severe pain, and weaker for mild or chronic pain. Use Moving Cupping up and down the side of chest for lateral chest pain.

UPPER BACK AND SCAPULAR PAIN

Upper back and scapular pain often coincide with neck and shoulder pain, which radiates down into the upper back and scapular region. Many of the causes of neck and shoulder pain also apply to upper back and scapular pain, as a lot of the muscles work together and affect each other, including poor posture and stress. Trauma and falls also cause upper back and scapular pain.

According to TCM, acute upper back pain is also an early sign of an infection, such as a cold or flu. This is due to pathogenic factors entering the channels of the neck and shoulder via Wind, blocking the movement of Qi and Blood. Sitting under an office vent that blows cold air can easily cause upper back pain.

GB21 *Jian Jing–Shoulder Well*

Location: On the most superior part of the shoulder, directly above the nipple, or halfway from the spine to the deltoid.

Affected muscles: Trapezius.

When to use: For upper back and shoulder pain. Used most often for stress-related upper back tension, working on the computer for too long, or achiness due to colds and flu.

Application: Apply Weak, Medium, or Strong Cupping for 10 to 15 minutes. Use stronger suction for acute or severe pain, and weaker for mild or chronic pain. Use Flash Cupping if upper back pain is due to a cold. Use Moving Cupping sideways across the trapezius muscle to loosen up the muscle and relieve upper back and scapular pain.

GV14 *Da Zhui–Great Hammer*

Location: Below the spinous process of the seventh cervical vertebra (C7), approximately level with the acromion (shoulders).

Affected muscles: Trapezius, rhomboid minor, serratus posterior superior.

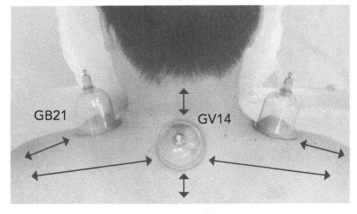

When to use: For upper back and shoulder pain. Used most often for stress-related upper back tension, working on the computer for too long, or achiness due to colds and flu. Used especially for burning upper back pain.

Application: Apply Weak, Medium, or Strong Cupping for 10 to 15 minutes. Use stronger suction for acute or severe pain, and weaker for mild or chronic pain. Use Flash Cupping if upper back pain is due to a cold. Use Moving Cupping up and down the spine, and sideways across the trapezius, to relieve tension in the upper back and scapular region. Use Bleeding Cupping on GV14 to relieve pain and inflammation quickly, especially if upper back or scapular pain has a burning sensation.

BL12 *Feng Men—Wind Gate*

Location: About 1.5 inches on either side of the spinous process of the second thoracic vertebra (T2).

Affected muscles: Trapezius, rhomboid minor, rhomboid major, erector spinae, semispinalis capitis, semispinalis cervicis, serratus posterior superior.

When to use: For upper back and shoulder pain. Used most often for stress-related upper back tension, working on the computer for too long, or achiness due to colds and flu.

Application: Apply Weak, Medium, or Strong Cupping for 10 to 15 minutes. Use stronger suction for acute or severe pain, and weaker for mild or chronic pain. Use Flash cupping if upper back or scapular pain is due to a cold. Use Moving

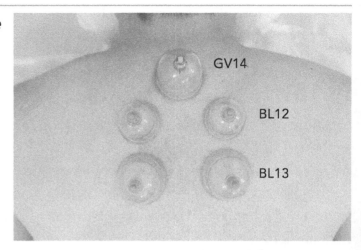

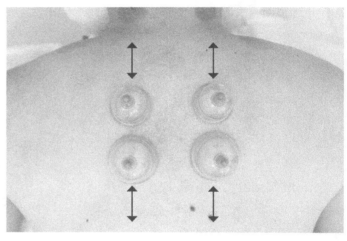

Cupping up and down the erector spinae to relieve pain in upper back and the area in between the scapulas.

BL13 *Fei Shu—Lung Shu*

Location: About 1.5 inches on either side of the spinous process of the third thoracic vertebra (T3).

Affected muscles: Trapezius, rhomboid minor, rhomboid major, erector spinae, semispinalis cervicis, semispinalis thoracis, serratus posterior superior.

When to use: For upper back and shoulder pain. Used most often for stress-related upper back tension, working on the computer for too long, or achiness due to colds and flu.

Application: Apply Weak, Medium, or Strong Cupping for 10 to 15 minutes. Use stronger suction for acute or severe pain, and weaker for mild or chronic pain. Use Flash cupping if upper back pain is due to a cold. Use Moving Cupping up and down the erector spinae to relieve the upper back and area in between the scapulas. Use Bleeding Cupping on BL13 to relieve upper back pain quickly.

BL15 *Xin Shu–Heart Shu*

Location: About 1.5 inches on either side of the spinous process of the fifth thoracic vertebra (T5).

Affected muscles: Trapezius, rhomboid minor, rhomboid major, erector spinae, semispinalis cervicis, semispinalis thoracis.

When to use: For upper back and shoulder pain. Used most often for stress-related upper back tension.

Application: Apply Weak, Medium, or Strong Cupping for 10 to 15 minutes. Use stronger suction for acute or severe pain, and weaker for mild or chronic pain. Use Flash cupping for upper back pain due to a cold. Use Moving Cupping up and down the erector spinae to relieve the upper back and area in between the scapulas. Use Bleeding Cupping on BL15 to relieve upper back pain quickly.

BL17 *Ge Shu–Diaphragm Shu*

Location: About 1.5 inches on either side of the spinous process of the seventh thoracic vertebra (T7).

Affected muscles: Trapezius, rhomboid minor, rhomboid major, erector spinae, semispinalis cervicis, semispinalis thoracis.

When to use: For upper back to mid-back pain.

Application: Apply Weak, Medium,

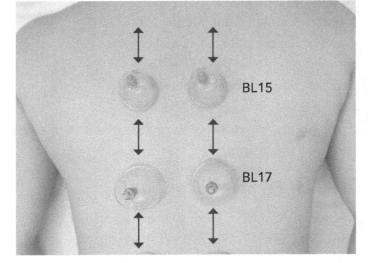

or Strong Cupping for 10 to 15 minutes. Use stronger suction for acute or severe pain, and weaker for mild or chronic pain. Use flash cupping for upper back pain due to a cold. Use Moving Cupping up and down the erector spinae to relieve the upper back and area in between the scapulas. Use Bleeding Cupping on BL17 to relieve upper back pain quickly.

SI11 *Tian Zong–Celestial Gathering*

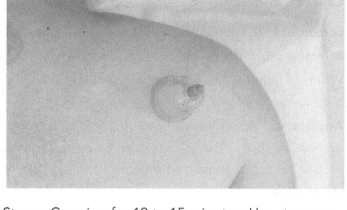

Location: On the scapula, in the depression in the center of the scapula, more specifically in the center of the subscapular fossa.

Affected muscles: Subscapularis, teres minor.

When to use: Used for scapular pain.

Application: Apply Weak, Medium, or Strong Cupping for 10 to 15 minutes. Use stronger suction for acute or severe pain, and weaker for mild or chronic pain. Use Flash Cupping if upper back or scapular pain is due to a cold. Apply Moving Cupping around the scapula to relieve shoulder and upper back pain. Use Bleeding Cupping on SI11 to relieve upper back pain quickly.

LOWER BACK PAIN

The lower back, or lumbar region, is prone to injury from sports, weight lifting, or carrying heavy objects, all of which often cause muscle strain. Cupping is an effective way to relieve strain and relax the muscles. Cupping can also be used to relieve the inflammation of sciatica, but it may have to be done gently, as the area will be very painful. When sciatica is caused by an inflamed piriformis (and includes shooting pain down the buttocks and into the legs), cupping can help to relieve the inflammation. This type of pain may require strong cupping, as the piriformis is deep in the buttocks.

Degenerative disc disorder causes chronic back pain. In TCM, the lumbar spine is governed by the Kidneys, which also govern the bones and joints. Gentle cupping can help replenish the Kidneys and the lumbar by bringing them fresh blood and nutrients to prevent degeneration. Sitting at a desk with poor posture all day can also cause lower back pain, as can unbalanced weight from carrying a bag or briefcase, especially if you tend to carry it over one shoulder.

If you have lower back pain with symptoms such as loss of bowel or bladder control, weakness in the legs, fever, or pain when coughing, you should consult a doctor. These symptoms may indicate something more serious and are most likely not due to a musculoskeletal issue.

GV4 *Shen Shu–Kidney Shu*

Location: In the space below the spinous process of the second lumbar vertebra (L2).

Affected muscles: Erector spinae, interspinales, multifidus, serratus posterior inferior.

When to use: For lower back pain that is right down the spine. Used for degenerative disc disorder and bulged disc.

Application: Apply Weak, Medium, or Strong Cupping for 10 to 15 minutes. Use stronger suction for acute or severe pain, and weaker for mild or chronic pain. DO NOT use strong suction on a person with a herniated disk. Use Flash Cupping to relieve lower back pain faster. Apply Moving Cupping up and down the erector spinae to relieve lower back pain, but don't be too aggressive over the spine, as it may hurt if the cups goes over the spine too fast or too hard.

BL23 *Shen Shu–Kidney Shu*

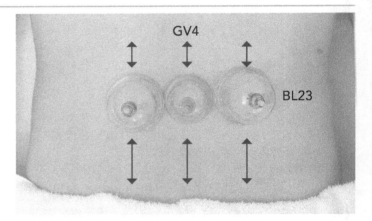

Location: About 1.5 inches on either side of the spinous process of the second lumbar vertebra (L2).

Affected muscles: Erector spinae, multifidus, quadratus lumborum, latissimus dorsi, serratus posterior inferior.

When to use: For lower back pain that is next to the spine, where the paraspinal muscles are. Used for sprained back and achy lower back from sitting or poor posture.

Application: Apply Weak, Medium, or Strong Cupping for 10 to 15 minutes. Use stronger suction for acute or severe pain, and weaker for mild or chronic pain. Use Flash Cupping to relieve lower back pain faster. Apply Moving Cupping up and down the erector spinae to relieve lower back pain, and Bleeding Cupping to relieve lower back pain quickly.

BL52 *Zhi Shi–Will Chamber*

Location: About 1.5 inches lateral to the BL23.

Affected muscles: Erector spinae, quadratus lumborum, latissimus dorsi, serratus posterior inferior.

When to use: For lower back pain that is more on the sides, lateral to the paraspinal muscles. Used for sprained back, and achy lower back from sitting or poor posture.

Application: Apply Weak, Medium, or Strong Cupping for 10 to 15 minutes. Use stronger suction for acute or severe pain, and weaker for mild or chronic pain. Use Flash Cupping to relieve lower back pain faster. Apply Moving Cupping up and down the latissimus dorsi or quadratus lumborum to relieve lower back pain that is on the side of the lower back.

BL25 *Da Chang Shu–Large Intestine Shu*

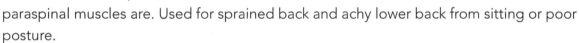

Location: About 1.5 inches on either side of the spinous process of the fourth lumbar vertebra (L4).

Affected muscles: Erector spinae, multifidus, quadratus lumborum, latissimus dorsi.

When to use: For lower back pain that is next to the spine, where the paraspinal muscles are. Used for sprained back and achy lower back from sitting or poor posture.

Application: Apply Weak, Medium, or Strong Cupping for 10 to 15 minutes. Use stronger suction for acute or severe pain, and weaker for mild or chronic pain. Use Flash Cupping to relieve lower back pain faster. Apply Moving Cupping up and down the erector spinae to relieve lower back pain, and Bleeding Cupping to relieve lower back pain quickly.

Yao Yan *Lumbar Eyes*

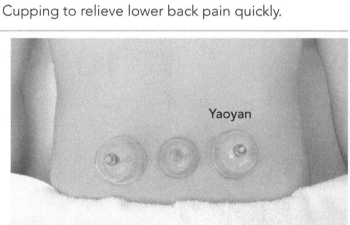

Yaoyan

Location: Approximately 3 to 4 inches on either side of the fourth lumbar vertebra (L4), or where the dimples just above the buttocks are located.

Affected muscles: Gluteus medius, gluteus maximus.

When to use: For lower back pain that radiates down into the gluteal muscles. Used for sprained back, and achy lower back from sitting or poor posture.

Application: Apply Medium or Strong Cupping for 10 to 15 minutes. Use stronger suction for acute or severe pain, and weaker for mild or chronic pain. Since there is a lot of muscle

and fat in this area, Weak Cupping may not be very effective. Use Flash cupping to relieve lower back, sciatica, or buttock pain faster. Apply Moving Cupping up and down the gluteus maximus or medius muscles to relieve lower back pain and sciatica.

BL53 *Bao Huang—Bladder Huang*

Location: Approximately 3 to 4 inches beside the second sacral foramen (S2), or 2 inches below Yao Yan.

Affected muscles: Gluteus maximus, gluteus medius.

When to use: For lower back pain that radiates down into the gluteal muscles. Used for sprained back, and achy lower back from sitting or poor posture.

Application: Apply Medium or Strong Cupping for 10 to 15 minutes. Use stronger suction for acute or severe pain, and weaker for mild or chronic pain. Since there is a lot of muscle and fat in this area, Weak Cupping may not be very effective. Use Flash Cupping to relieve lower back, sciatica, or buttock pain faster. Apply Moving Cupping up and down or across the gluteus maximus or medius muscles to relieve lower back pain and sciatica.

THIGH PAIN

Most types of thigh pain generally come from sports injuries. Most thigh injuries are acute but can become chronic if not treated or not treated properly.

The hamstrings, a group of three muscles made up of the semimembranosus, semitendinosus, and biceps femoris, are located at the back of the thigh. Sports injuries, especially those that involve a lot of running, are common here. The most common are muscle cramping due to not stretching before or after exercise, extensive use, or random muscle spasm. Many athletes routinely tear or strain their hamstrings.

The quads, or quadriceps femoris, which consist of the rectus femoris, vastus lateralis, vastus intermedius, and vastus medialis, are located at the front of the thigh. They are responsible for extending the knee and are important for standing, walking, climbing stairs, and running.

Just like the hamstrings, they are also easily injured in sports that involve a lot of running. The quadriceps can also be injured if you lift something too heavy.

Between the hamstrings and the quadriceps, the iliotibial, or IT band, lies on the side of the thigh and joins the hip and the knee. This ligament can get tight or injured by walking, running, or going up and down stairs a lot. It can also get tight if you sit too much, especially if you cross your legs when you sit.

Pain in the thigh can also be due to a referral pain from the lower back, such as the sciatica. The sciatic nerve runs through the thigh, and if the sciatic nerve is compressed or inflamed, it can cause shooting pain down the thighs.

ST32 *Fu Tu–Crouching Rabbit*

Location: Front of the thigh, about a third of the distance from the superior-lateral corner of the patella to the hip joint.

Affected muscles: Vastus lateralis, rectus femoris, vastus intermedius.

When to use: For pain of the lateral quadriceps muscles on the front of the thigh.

Application: Apply Medium or Strong Cupping for 10 to 15 minutes. Use stronger suction for acute or severe pain, and weaker for mild or chronic pain. Since there is a lot of muscle and fat in this area, Weak Cupping may not be very effective. Use Flash Cupping to relieve thigh pain faster, and Moving Cupping up and down the quads to relieve pain from the front of the thigh.

ST33 *Yin Shi–Yin Market*

Location: Front of the thigh, about four fingers' width (or approximately 3 inches) above the superior-lateral corner of the patella, or approximately 1 inch above ST34.

Affected muscles: Vastus lateralis, rectus femoris, vastus intermedius.

When to use: For pain of the lateral quadriceps muscles on the front of the thigh.

Application: Apply Medium or Strong Cupping for 10 to 15 minutes. Use stronger suction for acute or severe pain, and weaker for mild or chronic pain. Since there is a lot of muscle and fat in this area, Weak Cupping may not be very effective. Use Flash Cupping to relieve thigh pain faster, and Moving Cupping up and down the quadriceps muscles to relieve pain from the front of the thigh.

ST34 *Liang Qiu–Ridge Mound*

Location: Front of the thigh, three fingers' width (or approximately 2 inches) above the superior-lateral corner of the patella.

Affected muscles: Vastus lateralis.

When to use: For pain of the lateral quadriceps muscles on the front of the thigh.

Application: Apply Weak, Medium, or Strong Cupping for 10 to 15 minutes. Use stronger suction for acute or severe pain, and weaker for mild or chronic pain. Use Flash Cupping to relieve the thigh pain faster.

SP10 *Xue Hai–Sea of Blood*

Location: Front of the thigh, about three fingers' width (or approximately 2 inches) above the superior-medial corner of the patella.

Affected muscles: Vastus medialis.

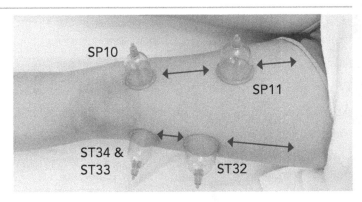

When to use: For pain of the medial quadriceps muscles on the front of the thigh.

Application: Apply Medium or Strong Cupping for 10 to 15 minutes. Use stronger suction for acute or severe pain, and weaker for mild or chronic pain. Since there is a lot of muscle and fat in this area, Weak Cupping may not be very effective. Use Flash Cupping to relieve thigh pain faster, and Moving Cupping up and down the quadriceps muscles to relieve pain from the front of the thigh.

SP11 *Ji Men–Winnower Gate*

Location: Front of the thigh, about a third of the distance from the superior-medial corner of the patella to the hip.

Affected muscles: Vastus medialis, sartorius.

When to use: For pain of the medial quadriceps muscles on the front of the thigh.

Application: Apply Medium or Strong Cupping for 10 to 15 minutes. Use stronger suction for acute or severe pain, and weaker for mild or chronic pain. Since there is a lot of muscle

and fat in this area, Weak Cupping may not be very effective. Use Flash Cupping to relieve the thigh pain faster, and Moving Cupping up and down the quadriceps muscles to relieve pain from the front of the thigh.

GB31 *Feng Shi–Wind Market*

Location: Side of the thigh, about a third of the distance from above the lateral end of the transverse popliteal crease (knee crease) to the greater trochanter of the femur.

Affected muscles: Biceps femoris, iliotibial band, vastus lateralis.

When to use: For pain that is on the iliotibial band on the sides of the thigh.

Application: Apply Weak, Medium, or Strong Cupping for 10 to 15 minutes. Use stronger suction for acute or severe pain, and weaker for mild or chronic pain. Use Flash Cupping to relieve thigh pain faster, and Moving Cupping up and down the iliotibial band to relieve pain from the side of the thigh.

GB33 *Xi Yang Guan–Knee Yang Gate*

Location: Side of the thigh, about three fingers' width (or approximately 2 inches) above the lateral end of the transverse popliteal crease (knee crease).

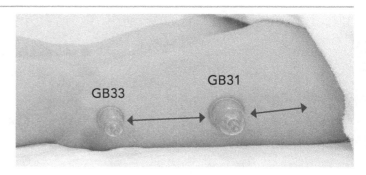

Affected muscles: Biceps femoris, iliotibial band, vastus lateralis.

When to use: For pain that is on the iliotibial band on the sides of the thigh.

Application: Apply Weak, Medium, or Strong Cupping for 10 to 15 minutes. Use stronger suction for acute or severe pain, and weaker for mild or chronic pain. Use Flash Cupping to relieve thigh pain faster, and Moving Cupping up and down the iliotibial band to relieve pain from the side of the thigh.

BL40 *Wei Zhong–Bend Middle*

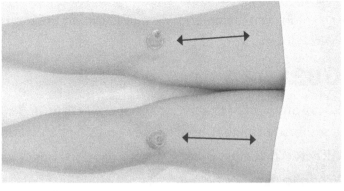

Location: Middle of the popliteal crease (crease behind the knees).

Affected muscles:
Semimembranosus, biceps femoris.

When to use: For pain of the hamstrings on the back of the thigh.

Application: Apply Weak or Medium Cupping for 10 to 15 minutes. Use stronger suction for acute or severe pain, and weaker for mild or chronic pain. Use Flash Cupping to relieve thigh pain faster, and Moving Cupping up and down the hamstrings to relieve pain from the back of the thigh.

BL36 *Cheng Fu–Supporter*

Location: Back of the thigh, middle of the gluteal crease (crease where the buttocks meet the thigh).

Affected muscles: Gluteus maximus, semitendinosus, biceps femoris.

When to use: For pain of the hamstrings on the back of the thigh.

Application: Apply Medium or Strong Cupping for 10 to 15 minutes. Use stronger suction for acute or severe pain, and weaker for mild or chronic pain. Since there is a lot of muscle and fat in this area, Weak Cupping may not be very effective. Use Flash Cupping to relieve thigh pain faster, and Moving Cupping up and down the hamstrings to relieve pain from the back of the thigh.

BL37 *Yin Men–Gate of Abundance*

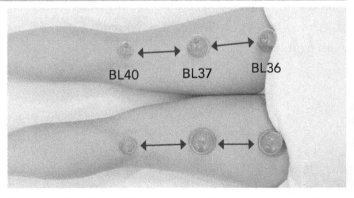

Location: Back of the thigh, about halfway between BL36 and BL40.

Affected muscles: Biceps femoris, semimembranosus, semitendinosus.

When to use: For pain of the hamstrings on the back of the thigh.

Application: Apply Medium or Strong Cupping for 10 to 15 minutes. Use stronger suction for acute or severe pain, and weaker for mild or chronic pain. Since there is a lot of muscle

and fat in this area, Weak Cupping may not be very effective. Use Flash Cupping to relieve thigh pain faster, and Moving Cupping up and down the hamstrings to relieve pain from the back of the thigh.

KNEE PAIN

Ligament tears and meniscus tears are among the most common sports injuries, and of these, an anterior cruciate ligament (ACL) injury is one of the most frequent. Other, less common ligament injuries can include the posterior cruciate ligament (PCL), lateral collateral ligament (LCL), and medial collateral ligament (MCL). Although cupping cannot fix any tears of the ligaments or menisci, it can help reduce pain and inflammation in the area. Tears need to be fixed with surgery, but after knee surgery, cupping can help bring fresh Qi, Blood, and nutrients to the area, at the same time break down scar tissue and clotted blood. Similarly, during recovery from fractures and dislocations, cupping can be useful to help reduce pain and inflammation, as well as bring fresh nutrients to help the area recover.

Arthritis of the knee is another frequent cause of knee pain. Rheumatoid arthritis is due to an autoimmune disease, which causes the body to attack the joints. Cupping can help clear inflammatory chemicals, which act as a signal for the body to attack the knee. Gouty arthritis is due to a buildup of uric acid in the body, which then crystallizes in and around joints, making them inflamed and painful. Cupping can help improve circulation, helping to drain uric acid from the area and reduce inflammation. Osteoarthritis is due to the wearing of the joints. Although nothing can be done to fix the joint once it has degraded, cupping can help prevent further damage by helping to reduce inflammation and pain in the area.

BL40 *Wei Zhong–Bend Middle*

Location: Middle of the popliteal crease (crease behind the knees).

Affected muscles:
Semimembranosus, biceps femoris, plantaris, gastrocnemius.

When to use: For knee pain that is in the back of the knees.

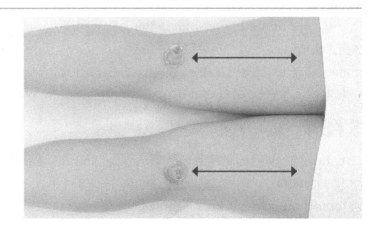

Application: Apply Weak or Medium Cupping for 10 to 15 minutes. Use stronger suction for acute or severe pain, and weaker for mild or chronic pain. Use Flash Cupping to relieve knee pain faster. , and Moving Cupping up and down the hamstrings.

SP10 *Xue Hai—Sea of Blood*

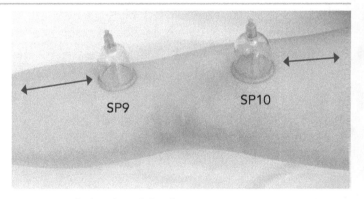

Location: About three fingers' width (or approximately 2 inches) above the superior-medial corner of the patella.

Affected muscles: Vastus medialis.

When to use: For knee pain that is in the front of the knees, above the knees, or medial side of the knees.

Application: Apply Weak, Medium, or Strong Cupping for 10 to 15 minutes. Use stronger suction for acute or severe pain, and weaker for mild or chronic pain. Use Flash Cupping to relieve knee pain faster, and Moving Cupping up and down the quadriceps muscles.

SP9 *Yin Ling Quan—Yin Mound Spring*

Location: In the depression just below and behind the medial condyle of the tibia.

Affected muscles: Gastrocnemius, soleus.

When to use: For knee pain that is in the front of the knees, below the knees, or medial side of the knees.

Application: Apply Weak, Medium, or Strong Cupping for 10 to 15 minutes. Use stronger suction for acute or severe pain, and weaker for mild or chronic pain. Use Flash Cupping to relieve the knee pain faster, and Moving Cupping up and down the front of the leg.

ST34 *Liang Qiu—Ridge Mound*

Location: Three fingers' width (or approximately 2 inches) above the superior-lateral corner of the patella.

Affected muscles: Vastus lateralis.

When to use: For knee pain that is in the front of the knees, above the knees, or lateral side of the knees.

Application: Apply Weak, Medium, or Strong Cupping for 10 to 15 minutes. Use stronger suction for acute or severe pain, and weaker for mild or chronic pain. Use Flash Cupping and Moving Cupping to relieve the knee pain faster.

ST36 *Zu San Li—Leg Three Miles*

Location: Four fingers' width (or approximately 3 inches) below the inferior-lateral corner of the patella, and a thumb's width (or 1 inch) lateral to the tibia (shinbone).

Affected muscles: Tibialis anterior, extensor digitorum longus.

When to use: For knee pain that

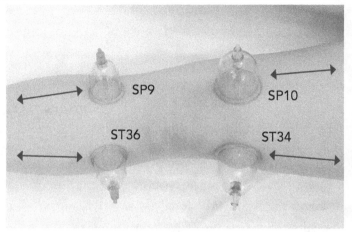

is in the front of the knees, below the knees, or lateral side of the knees. Can be used for pain, tightness, or weakness on any part of the leg.

Application: Apply Weak, Medium, or Strong Cupping for 10 to 15 minutes. Use stronger suction for acute or severe pain, and weaker for mild or chronic pain. Use Flash Cupping and Moving Cupping to relieve knee pain faster.

Heding *Crane's Summit*

Location: In the depression directly above the middle of the upper border of the patella (kneecap).

Affected muscles: Rectus femoris, vastus intermedius.

When to use: For knee pain that is in the front of the knees, and above the knees.

Application: Apply Weak, Medium, or Strong Cupping for 10 to 15 minutes. Use stronger suction for acute or severe pain, and weaker for mild or chronic pain. Use Flash Cupping to relieve knee pain faster.

LOWER LEG PAIN

A major cause of lower leg pain is frequent walking or running, or activities that involve a lot of either action. People often wear shoes without proper ankle and arch support. Without this, twisting the ankle and other injuries can occur more easily. Uncomfortable shoes also cause you to walk improperly, which can ruin your walking posture, cause your whole body to become misaligned, and cause all sorts of joint or muscle pain, or, if the misalignment is severe, injury.

A common lower leg injury is to strain the calf muscle (gastrocnemius), usually due to exercise or sports. It is important to stretch before and after exercise to prevent injury. The Achilles tendon, which attaches your gastrocnemius to your heel, can also get injured easily if you don't stretch, possibly leading to tendonitis or tear, and heel or foot pain.

Leg cramps are another type of lower leg pain that can be caused by overexercising, not drinking enough water, losing electrolytes from excessive sweating, or not stretching before and after exercise. In TCM, cramps are a common symptom in people who have anemia. Since the lower leg is so far from the heart and there is not enough blood in the body to nourish the muscles in the lower leg, they become malnourished and can tighten suddenly, causing cramps.

BL40 *Wei Zhong–Bend Middle*

Location: Middle of the popliteal crease (crease behind the knees).

Affected muscles: Semimembranosus, biceps femoris, plantaris, gastrocnemius, popliteus.

When to use: For calf pain or tightness.

Application: Apply Weak or Medium Cupping for 10 to 15 minutes. Use stronger suction for acute or severe

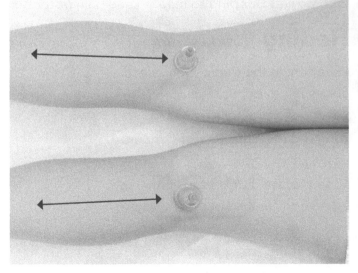

pain, and weaker for mild or chronic pain. Use Moving Cupping up and down the calf to help relieve calf pain, and Flash Cupping to relieve the calf pain faster.

BL57 *Cheng San–Mountain Support*

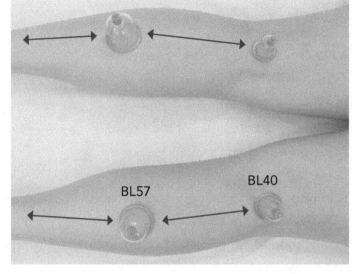

Location: Halfway between the knee and the ankle, in between the two heads of the gastrocnemius muscle.

Affected muscles: Gastrocnemius, soleus, tibialis posterior, flexor digitorum longus, flexor hallucis longus, plantaris.

When to use: For calf pain or tightness.

Application: Apply Weak, Medium, or Strong Cupping for 10 to 15 minutes. Use stronger suction for acute or severe pain, and weaker for mild or chronic pain. Use Moving Cupping up and down the calf to help relieve calf pain, and Flash Cupping to relieve the calf pain faster.

ST36 *Zu San Li–Leg Three Miles*

Location: Four fingers' width (or approximately 3 inches) below the inferior-lateral corner of the patella, and a thumb's width (or 1 inch) lateral to the tibia (shin bone).

Affected muscles: Tibialis anterior, extensor digitorum longus.

When to use: For pain or tightness of the muscles just lateral to the shin bone. Can be used for pain, tightness, or weakness on any part of the leg.

Application: Apply Weak, Medium, or Strong Cupping for 10 to 15 minutes. Use stronger suction for acute or severe pain, and weaker for mild or chronic pain. Use Moving Cupping up and down the anterior part of the leg to help with lower leg pain, and Flash Cupping to relieve lower leg pain faster.

ST39 *Xia Ju Xu–Lower Great Hollow*

Location: One thumb's width (or approximately 1 inch) below the midpoint of the inferior-lateral corner of the patella to the ankle.

Affected muscles: Tibialis anterior, extensor digitorum longus, extensor hallucis longus.

When to use: For pain or tightness of the muscles just lateral to the shin bone.

Application: Apply Weak, Medium, or Strong Cupping for 10 to 15 minutes. Use stronger suction for acute or severe pain, and weaker for mild or chronic pain. Use Moving Cupping up and down the anterior part of the leg to help with lower leg pain, and Flash Cupping to relieve the lower leg pain faster.

GB34 *Yang Ling Quan– Yang Mound Spring*

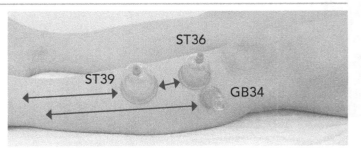

Location: In the depression anterior and inferior to the head of the fibula.

Affected muscles: Fibularis longus, fibularis brevis.

When to use: For pain or tightness of the muscles on the side of the lower leg, and muscles along the fibula.

Application: Apply Weak, Medium, or Strong Cupping for 10 to 15 minutes. Use stronger suction for acute or severe pain, and weaker for mild or chronic pain. Use Moving Cupping up and down the lateral part of the leg to help with lower leg pain, and Flash Cupping to relieve the lower leg pain faster.

ANKLE PAIN

The most common cause of ankle pain is twisting or rolling your ankle, resulting in a sprain. A sprain is an injury to the ligaments, which connect one bone to another bone. When you roll or twist your ankle, it can stretch or even tear the ligament. There are two main types of ankle sprains: eversion and inversion. An inversion, or lateral ankle sprain, happens when you roll the outside of your foot, and an eversion, or medial ankle sprain, happens when you roll the inside of your foot. If the sprain is severe, it may even cause a fracture of one of the bones in the joint. Spraining your ankle once can cause you to sprain it more easily in the future. To prevent this, make sure you wear comfortable shoes that fit and have proper ankle and arch support. People who have flat feet or high arches can sprain their ankles more easily and need proper orthotic pads to correct their arch.

GB40 *Qiu Xu–Hill Ruins*

Location: In the depression anterior and inferior to the lateral malleolus.

Affected tendon/ligament: Fibularis longus, fibularis brevis.

When to use: For lateral ankle pain, sprain, or strain.

Application: Apply Weak or Medium Cupping for 10 to 15 minutes. There is not a lot of flesh in this area, so do not use Strong Cupping.

BL62 *Shen Mai–Extending Vessel*

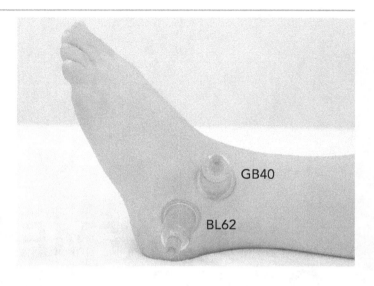

Location: In the depression directly below the lateral malleolus.

Affected tendon/ligament: Fibularis longus, fibularis brevis.

When to use: For lateral ankle pain, sprain, or strain.

Application: Apply Weak or Medium Cupping for 10 to 15 minutes. There is not a lot of flesh in this area, so do not use Strong Cupping.

SP5 *Shang Qiu–Shang Hill*

Location: In the depression anterior and inferior to the medial malleolus.

Affected tendon/ligament: Tibialis anterior.

When to use: For medial ankle pain, sprain, or strain.

Application: Apply Weak or Medium Cupping for 10 to 15 minutes. There is not a lot of flesh in this area, so do not use Strong Cupping.

K16 *Zhao Hai–Shining Sea*

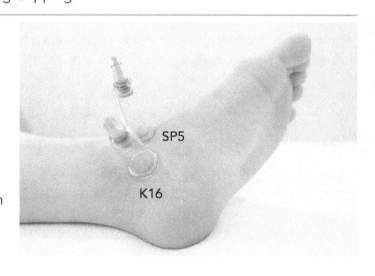

Location: In the depression directly below the medial malleolus.

Affected tendon/ligament: Tibialis anterior.

When to use: For medial ankle pain, sprain, or strain.

Application: Apply Weak or Medium Cupping for 10 to 15 minutes. There is not a lot of flesh in this area, so do not use Strong Cupping.

CHAPTER 6

TREATMENT OF OTHER CONDITIONS

Cupping is not only used for pain in TCM. It is one of the primary modalities used by practitioners to treat almost any disease. Disease happens when there is an imbalance in the body, when a pathogen invades, or when one of the organs does not work properly or efficiently. Cupping can help restore balance to the body, remove pathogens and toxins, and regulate and nourish the internal organs. While it may not be able to cure your disease, it can help it, depending on what the cause is.

Here I will list some common, everyday ailments that cupping can help alleviate, assuming the symptoms or the cause is not very serious. I will discuss anti-aging and beauty issues, digestion, gynecological trouble, respiratory issues, infections, and psychological issues.

If the symptoms of these conditions are serious or do not alleviate after a couple of days, please see your healthcare practitioner for a proper diagnosis. This book is not for self-diagnosing your disease. There are many causes of each disease that cupping may not be effective for, or for which a highly trained practitioner of cupping would be needed to produce effective results, so please see your healthcare practitioner if you have any questions.

CELLULITE

Cellulite, the dimpling of the skin caused by the uneven distribution of fat tissues, is not a disease—it's normal and very common. It usually occurs in areas where there tends to be more fat such as the thighs, buttocks, hips, abdomen, arms, or breasts. The older we get, the more likely we are to get cellulite because the skin loses its elasticity.

Cupping can be effective in treating cellulite. Cellulite may be due to poor lymphatic drainage, and Moving Cupping is excellent for lymphatic drainage. Fat travels through the body via the lymph, so helping to move the lymph can prevent fat deposit in an area. Cupping can also bring fresh Blood and nutrients to the area, which can help the skin become healthier and tighter. Cupping can also stimulate collagen formation, firming the skin and reducing the appearance of cellulite.

Treatment *Cellulite*

Location: Place the cups on the area where the cellulite is located, whether it is on the thighs, buttocks, hips, abdomen, arms, or breasts. There are no specific points for cellulite.

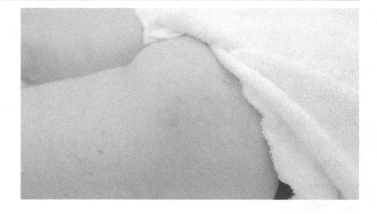

Application: Use Moving Cupping on the area where the cellulite is located. Use light to medium suction for areas that are smaller, bonier, or have less muscle and fat, and stronger suction for those that are larger and have more muscle and fat. Your intention is not to get any bruise marks, but rather to break down the fat. Move the cups around with a moderate speed for 5 minutes per area. This can be done

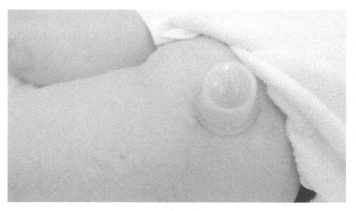

every day, and results can be immediate, but lasting effects may take two to three weeks, depending on the severity of the cellulite.

STRETCH MARKS

Stretch marks are lines that appear when the body is growing faster than the skin can, so the skin breaks and forms scar-like tissues. They appear over areas that tend to experience rapid weight gain or rapid weight loss, most commonly the abdomen, breasts, hips, buttocks, and thighs. They are common during and after pregnancy, when women experience rapid weight gain. During puberty, stretch marks can result from periods of rapid growth. Stretch marks are natural, but some people may feel they are unsightly and may be self-conscious of them. Cupping can help break down the scarring that forms the stretch marks, improve blood circulation, and increase collagen production.

Treatment *Stretch Marks*

Location: Place the cups on the area where you have stretch marks, whether it is on the abdomen, breasts, hips, buttocks, or thighs. There are no specific points for stretch marks.

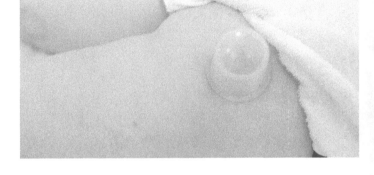

Application: Use Moving Cupping on the area where the stretch marks are located. Use light to medium suction for areas that are smaller, bonier, or have less muscle and fat, and stronger suction for those that are larger and have more muscle and fat. Your intention is not to get any bruise marks, but rather to break down the scar tissue that makes up the stretch mark. Move the cups in a circular motion on top of the stretch marks for 5 minutes per area. This can be done every day, and results can be immediate, but lasting effects may take two to three weeks, depending on the severity of the stretch marks.

ANTI-AGING/WRINKLES

Throughout history, people, both male and female, have wanted to look younger. Most anti-aging and beauty products are marketed toward women, but the male anti-aging industry is growing rapidly. According to TCM, aging is a natural process, one your lifestyle, diet, and health can affect. The main organ responsible for growing and development is the Kidneys, so activity or food that taxes the Kidneys will accelerate aging.

The causes of wrinkles all come down to the body, specifically the skin, being able to regenerate itself. As we age, the skin's supporting structures, collagen and connective tissue, regenerate more slowly, so the skin starts to lose elasticity and sag, creating wrinkles.

Cupping can be used to not only smooth out the wrinkles, but also bring blood flow and nutrients to the skin cells, helping them make more collagen, which can reduce wrinkles over time. Cupping can also help the body's overall health improve, which can help the skin look more youthful and healthy.

Treatment *Anti-Aging and Wrinkles*

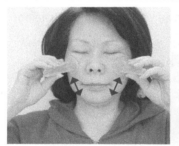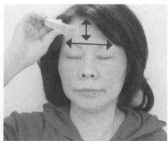
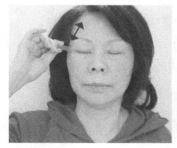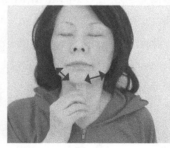

Location: Place the cups on the areas of the face or body where you have wrinkles. There are no specific points for wrinkles.

Application: Use Moving Cupping on the area where the wrinkles are located. Generally, special facial cups are used, which are small silicone cups. Use light suction for areas of the face. Use slightly stronger suction for other areas of the body. Your intention is not to get any bruise marks, but rather to bring nutrients to the area and to help collagen build up. Move the cups in a circular motion on top of the wrinkles for 5 minutes per area. This can be done every day, and results can be immediate, but lasting effects may take two to three weeks, depending on your age and how deep your wrinkles are.

ABDOMINAL BLOATING

Bloating refers to a sense of fullness, which can cause mild to severe discomfort. It tends to happen in the upper abdomen (epigastrium) where your stomach is, the lower abdomen (hypogastrium), or the entire abdomen. Acute episodes tend to happen if you eat too much, particularly of a certain type of food or a food you have intolerance to. Chronic or severe bloating is often uncomfortable and annoying, causing poor appetite or nausea, at which time it is best to seek professional help.

Abdominal bloating can be due to a weak digestive system, overeating, food intolerances or allergies, gastritis (the inflammation of the lining of the stomach), and constipation (see page 74 for more information).

CV12 *Zhong Wan—Central Stomach*

Location: On the anterior midline of the body, halfway between the sternum and umbilicus.

When to use: Good for most types of bloating around the stomach area, as it helps to improve digestion and move food along the digestive tract.

Application: Use Weak to Medium Cupping for 10 to 15 minutes. Apply Moving Cupping in a clockwise direction to help move gas, food, and waste along the digestive tract.

CV6 *Qi Hai—Sea of Qi*

Location: On the anterior midline of the body, around a thumb's length (or 1.5 inches) below the umbilicus.

When to use: For bloating around the lower abdomen. Helps move things in the lower abdomen and improve the body as a whole.

Application: Use Weak to Medium Cupping for 10 to 15 minutes. Apply Moving Cupping in a clockwise direction to help move gas, food, and waste along the digestive tract.

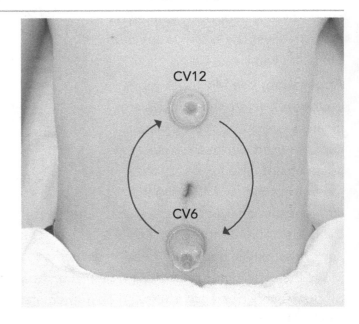

ST25 *Tian Shu–Celestial Pivot*

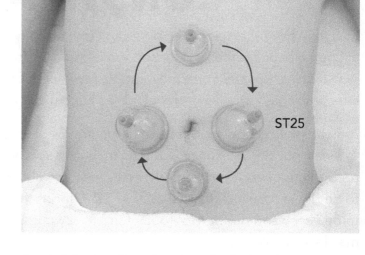

Location: Around three fingers' breadth (or approximately 2 inches) on either side of the umbilicus.

When to use: For any type of bloating, or bloating of the abdomen as a whole. Especially effective if constipation is causing the bloating as it helps to promote bowel movement.

Application: Apply Weak to Medium Cupping for 10 to 15 minutes. Apply Moving Cupping in a clockwise direction to help move gas, food, and waste along the digestive tract.

BL20 *Pi Shu–Spleen Shu*

Location: 1.5 inches on either side of the spinous process of the eleventh thoracic vertebra (T11).

When to use: For any type of bloating, and to strengthen the digestive system.

Application: Use Medium Cupping for 10 to 15 minutes. Apply Moving Cupping in a downward direction to help move the digestive tract.

BL25 *Da Chang Shu–Large Intestine Shu*

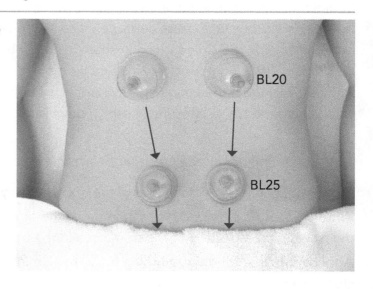

Location: 1.5 inches on either side of the spinous process of the fourth lumbar vertebra (L4).

When to use: For bloating due to constipation. Helps to promote bowel movement.

Application: Use Medium Cupping for 10 to 15 minutes. Apply Moving Cupping in a downward direction to help move the digestive tract.

CONSTIPATION

Everyone has suffered from constipation (the inability to pass stools for more than two days) at one point or another, but for some, it is chronic, often occurring for years or even decades. Acute cases, such as from dehydration, fever, or eating a certain food, are usually resolved after a few days. However, chronic cases are difficult and stubborn to fix.

A diet high in protein and fat and low in fiber is often the cause of constipation. Fiber helps to clean out the intestines and add bulk to stools, while fats and proteins slow down the transit time of waste through the intestines, so more water is absorbed, causing the stools to be dry and difficult to push out. In TCM, foods that are high in fats and proteins are said to be very warm or hot. Hot foods tend to dry out the body, which is why eating spicy food may lead to constipation. Not drinking enough water or taking large quantities of diuretic substances, such as coffee or soda, can promote excessive urination, which can also dry your body and intestines out, leading to constipation.

Lack of exercise also contributes to constipation. Exercise, especially aerobic or cardio exercise, causes us to breathe a lot faster. The up-and-down movement of the diaphragm when we breathe actually helps move the bowels. In TCM, the Lungs and the Large Intestines are paired organs. The Lungs help the Large Intestine function by pushing Qi downward. Pushing the stools out of the body needs a downward movement of Qi. So, if you have weak Lungs, you may have constipation as a result.

Sometimes, stressful situations such as traveling lead people to experience constipation. In TCM, this is because stress negatively affects the Liver, which moves Qi throughout your body and helps the Spleen in digestion. When you are stressed, the Liver cannot move Qi properly, causing your bowels to move more slowly. Other emotions, such as grief or sadness, can affect the Lungs in TCM. Again, when the Lungs are negatively affected, they cannot help the Large Intestines push Qi downward.

CV12 *Zhong Wan—Central Stomach*

Location: On the anterior midline of the body, halfway between the sternum and umbilicus.

When to use: As a general point to improve the digestive system. Can help move the digestive tract, especially of the stomach and the transverse colon.

Application: Use Medium Cupping for 10 to 15 minutes. Apply Moving Cupping in a clockwise direction to help waste along the digestive tract and promote bowel movement.

CV6 *Qi Hai–Sea of Qi*

Location: On the anterior midline of the body, around a thumb's length (or 1.5 inches) below the umbilicus.

When to use: To move things in the lower abdomen and promote bowel movement.

Application: Use Medium Cupping for 10 to 15 minutes. Apply Moving Cupping in a clockwise direction to help move the digestive tract and promote bowel movement.

ST25 *Tian Shu–Celestial Pivot*

Location: Around three fingers' breadth (or approximately 2 inches) on either side of the umbilicus.

When to use: For any large intestine problem, to regulate the bowels and promote bowel movement.

Application: Use Medium Cupping for 10 to 15 minutes. Apply Moving Cupping in a clockwise direction to help move the digestive tract and promote bowel movement.

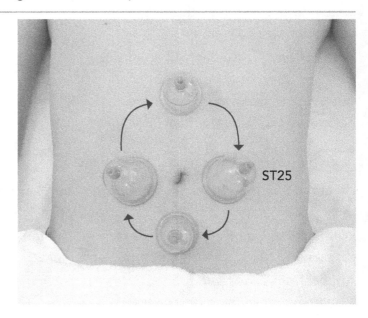

BL20 *Pi Shu–Spleen Shu*

Location: 1.5 inches on either side of spinous process of the eleventh thoracic vertebra (T11).

When to use: For any type of constipation, especially if there is no urge to have a bowel movement. Strengthens the digestive system, especially for slow peristalsis or slow digestive system.

Application: Use Medium Cupping for 10 to 15 minutes. Apply Moving Cupping in a downward direction to help move the digestive tract.

BL25 *Da Chang Shu– Large Intestine Shu*

Location: 1.5 inches on either side of the spinous process of the fourth lumbar vertebra (L4).

When to use: For any type of large intestine problem, this helps promote bowel movement.

Application: Use Medium Cupping for 10 to 15 minutes. Apply Moving Cupping in a downward direction to help move the digestive tract.

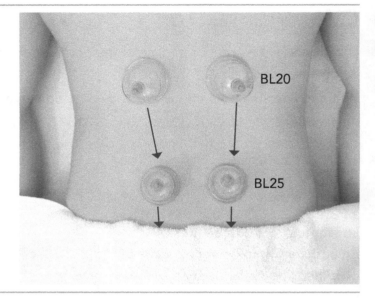

ST36 *Zu San Li–Leg Three Miles*

Location: Four fingers' width (or approximately 3 inches) below the lateral-inferior corner of the patella, and one thumb's width (about 1 inch) lateral to the tibia (shinbone).

When to use: To help improve the digestive system as a whole. Can help move the digestive system and promote bowel movement.

Application: Use Medium Cupping for 10 to 15 minutes. Apply Moving Cupping down the leg to help move the digestive tract.

ST37 *Shang Ju Xu–Upper Great Void*

Location: Four fingers' width (or approximately 3 inches) below ST36, and about one thumb's width (or 1 inch) lateral to the tibia (shinbone).

When to use: For any large intestine problem. Can help move the digestive system and promote bowel movement.

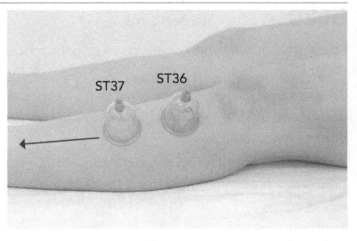

Application: Use Medium Cupping for 10 to 15 minutes. Apply Moving Cupping down the leg to help move the digestive tract.

DIARRHEA

Most diarrhea is short-lived, only occurring when someone is sick, eats something that disagrees with their digestive system, or eats something that is unclean. However, some people may suffer from diarrhea for many weeks, months, or even years. Diarrhea may be inconvenient or embarrassing, but in developing countries, it is very dangerous. Causes include the stomach flu, food poisoning, food intolerance (such as to dairy), irritable bowel syndrome (IBS), ulcerative colitis (UC), and Crohn's disease.

In TCM, the causes are often associated with a weak Spleen, the Liver, excessive Dampness attacking the Spleen, or eating too much Heating food.

CV12 *Zhong Wan–Central Stomach*

Location: On the anterior midline of the body, halfway between the sternum and umbilicus.

When to use: As a general point to improve the digestive system.

Application: Use Weak to Medium Cupping for 10 to 15 minutes. Apply Moving Cupping in a counterclockwise direction to slow down bowel movement and stop diarrhea.

CV6 *Qi Hai–Sea of Qi*

Location: On the anterior midline of the body, around one thumb's length (or 1.5 inches) below the umbilicus.

When to use: To strengthen the body as a whole. Especially useful if diarrhea is due to a weak digestive system.

Application: Use Weak to Medium Cupping for 10 to 15 minutes. Apply Moving Cupping in a counterclockwise direction to help slow down the digestive tract and stop diarrhea.

ST25 *Tian Shu–Celestial Pivot*

Location: Around three fingers' breadth (or approximately 2 inches) on either side of the umbilicus.

When to use: For any large intestine problem, helping to regulate the bowels, and stop diarrhea.

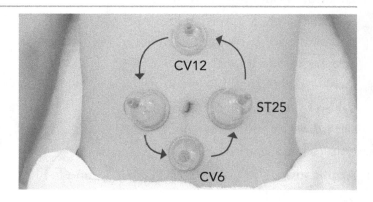

Application: Use Weak to Medium Cupping for 10 to 15 minutes. Apply Moving Cupping in a counterclockwise direction to help slow down the digestive tract and stop diarrhea.

BL20 *Pi Shu–Spleen Shu*

Location: 1.5 inches on either side of the spinous process of the eleventh thoracic vertebra (T11).

When to use: For any type of diarrhea, especially chronic loose stools. Strengthens the digestive system.

Application: Use Weak to Medium Cupping for 10 to 15 minutes. Apply Moving Cupping in an upward direction to help stop diarrhea.

BL25 *Da Chang Shu–Large Intestine Shu*

Location: 1.5 inches on either side of the spinous process of the fourth lumbar vertebra (L4).

When to use: For any type of large intestine problem. Helps to stop diarrhea.

Application: Use Weak to Medium Cupping for 10 to 15 minutes. Apply

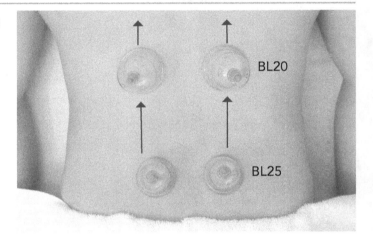

Moving Cupping in an upward direction to help stop diarrhea.

ST36 *Zu San Li–Leg Three Miles*

Location: Four fingers' width (or approximately 3 inches) below the lateral-inferior corner of the patella, and about one thumb's width (or 1 inch) lateral to the tibia (shinbone).

When to use: To help improve the digestive system as a whole. Can help to stop diarrhea.

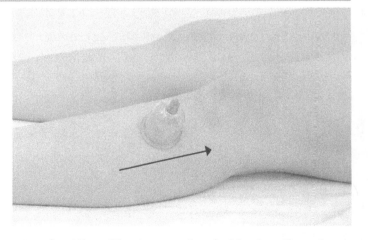

Application: Use Weak to Medium Cupping for 10 to 15 minutes. Apply Moving Cupping up the leg to help stop diarrhea.

ST37 *Shang Ju Xu– Upper Great Void*

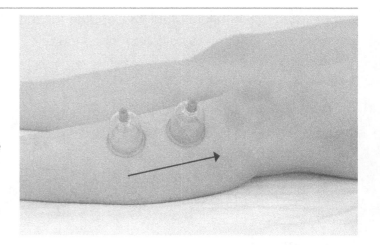

Location: Four fingers' width below ST36, and a thumb's width (about 1 inch) lateral to the tibia (shinbone).

When to use: For any large intestine problem. Can help stop diarrhea.

Application: Use Weak to Medium Cupping for 10 to 15 minutes. Apply Moving Cupping up the leg to help stop diarrhea.

POOR APPETITE

Poor appetite or loss of appetite is called anorexia (this is not to be confused with the eating disorder, anorexia nervosa). Most causes are relatively harmless, but some may be quite serious. Some of the main culprits are acute infection, pain, stress/emotions, chronic disease, poor/weak digestive system, metabolic disease, or side effects of medications.

According to TCM, poor appetite caused by acute infection is due to the Wind pathogen invading, and cupping can help suck the Wind pathogen out. For poor appetite due to pain, the cause is stagnation of Qi and Blood, and cupping is very good at moving the Qi and Blood, releasing the blockages, and stopping pain. Stress and emotions reduce the Liver's ability to send Qi and Blood to the Stomach and Spleen, making you lose your appetite; cupping can help to move the Qi and Blood in the body, soothe the Liver, and calm the mind. People with chronic disease or illness often have poor appetite; cupping can help boost the body's energy and strengthen the digestive system. Cupping can help strengthen a weak digestive system as well as move the digestive system faster, improving the appetite.

CV12 *Zhong Wan–Central Stomach*

Location: On the anterior midline of the body, halfway between the sternum and umbilicus.

When to use: As a general point to improve the digestive system and appetite.

Application: Use Weak to Medium Cupping for 10 to 15 minutes. Apply Moving Cupping in a clockwise direction to help promote digestion.

CV6 *Qi Hai—Sea of Qi*

Location: On the anterior midline of the body, around one thumb's length (or 1.5 inches) below the umbilicus.

When to use: To strengthen the body as a whole. Especially useful if have you a weak digestive system.

Application: Use Weak to Medium Cupping for 10 to 15 minutes. Apply Moving Cupping in a clockwise direction to help promote digestion.

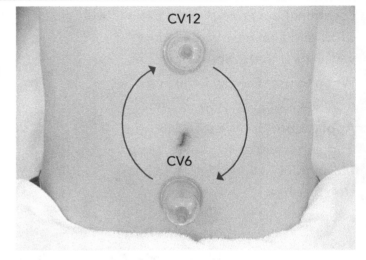

BL20 *Pi Shu—Spleen Shu*

Location: 1.5 inches on either side of the eleventh thoracic vertebra (T11).

When to use: As a general point to strengthen the digestive system, helping to increase appetite.

Application: Use Weak to Medium Cupping for 10 to 15 minutes.

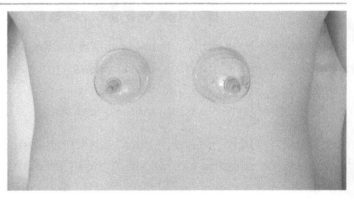

ST36 *Zu San Li—Leg Three Miles*

Location: Four fingers' width (or approximately 3 inches) below the inferior-lateral corner of the patella, and about one thumb's width (or 1 inch) lateral to the tibia (shinbone).

When to use: To help improve the digestive system as a whole, increasing appetite.

Application: Use Weak to Medium Cupping for 10 to 15 minutes.

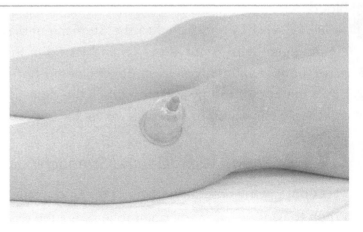

IRREGULAR MENSTRUATION

Irregular menstruation may indicate an imbalance in the body, such as a disharmony of estrogen and progesterone. This can be caused by going off birth control (which is made of estrogen and progesterone), polycystic ovarian syndrome (PCOS), thyroid problems, and uterine fibroids (polyps). Cupping can help regulate the bodily imbalances, which can lead to regular menstruation.

According to TCM, irregular menstruation may be due to working excessively and not getting enough rest, which can cause the body to become drained and weakened over time. When the Spleen weakens, it cannot control the flow of blood, causing it to escape early. Cupping can help strengthen the body and Spleen.

An irregular diet—such as not eating enough or eating meals that are not nutritious—can also damage and weaken the Spleen, causing early periods. Consuming too much food that is hot in nature, like spicy foods, can cause Heat to build up in the body. Heat makes blood flow faster and more recklessly, which makes it break out of the blood vessels easily, causing early periods. Cold foods, such as raw or refrigerated foods or drinks, can cause Cold to build up in the body, slowing down movement and delaying periods. Cupping can help strengthen the Spleen, as well as suck out the pathogenic Heat or Cold in the body.

Emotional stress, anger, or frustration can cause the Liver to work improperly. The Liver is said to move Qi throughout the body, and the Qi movement drives the flow of blood. Liver Blood is said to be the source of menstrual blood. If the Liver is stressed out, Qi and Blood do not flow, causing delayed menstruation. Cupping is very good at moving Qi and Blood, helping regulate menstruation.

Chronic illness can also cause the body to become weakened. This especially affects the Kidneys, which are said to be in charge of menstruation. So, if the Kidneys are weakened, menstruation becomes irregular. Cupping can help nourish and strengthen the Kidneys, helping them to regulate menstruation.

CV4 *Guan Yuan–Origin Pass*

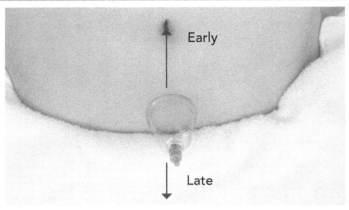

Location: On the anterior midline of the lower abdomen, three fingers' breadth (or approximately 2 inches) above the pubic bone.

When to use: For all types of irregular menstruation.

Application: Use Medium to Strong Cupping for 10 to 15 minutes. Apply Moving Cupping downward toward pubis if menstruation is late, and upward toward umbilicus a week before menstruation if menstruation usually comes early.

Zi Gong *Child Palace*

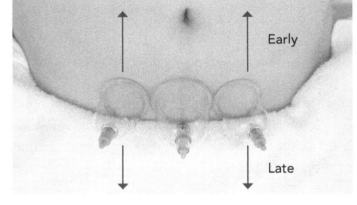

Location: Four fingers' breadth (or approximately 3 inches) lateral to and one thumb's width (or 1 inch) below CV4.

When to use: For all types of irregular menstruation.

Application: Use Medium to Strong Cupping for 10 to 15 minutes. Apply Moving Cupping downward toward pubis if menstruation is late, and upward toward umbilicus a week before menstruation if menstruation usually comes early.

SP10 *Xue Hai–Sea of Blood*

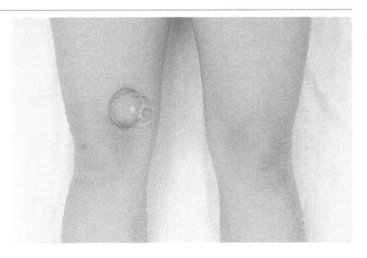

Location: Three fingers' width (or approximately 2 inches) medial and superior to the superior-medial corner of the patella.

When to use: To regulate the Blood, and for all types of irregular menstruation, but better for late periods with painful menstruation.

Application: Apply Medium to Strong Cupping for 10 to 15 minutes.

SP6 *San Yin Jiao–Three Yin Intersection*

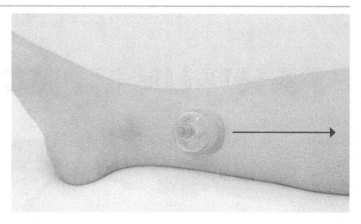

Location: Four fingers' breadth (or approximately 3 inches) above the tip of the medial malleolus, posterior to the medial border of the tibia.

When to use: For all types of irregular menstruation, but better for late periods.

Application: Use Weak, Medium, or Strong Cupping for 10 to 15 minutes. Apply Moving Cupping upward toward the knee if menstruation is late.

BL18 *Gan Shu–Liver Shu*

Location: 1.5 inches on either side of the spinous process of the ninth thoracic vertebra (T9).

When to use: For all types of irregular menstruation, but better for late periods with painful menstruation.

Application: Use Weak, Medium, or Strong Cupping for 10 to 15 minutes. Apply Moving Cupping down the back if menstruation is late, and up the back one week before menstruation if menstruation tends to be early.

BL23 *Shen Shu–Kidney Shu*

Location: About 1.5 inches on either side of the spinous process of the second lumbar vertebra (L2).

When to use: For all types of irregular menstruation.

Application: Use Weak, Medium, or Strong Cupping for 10 to 15 minutes. Apply Moving Cupping

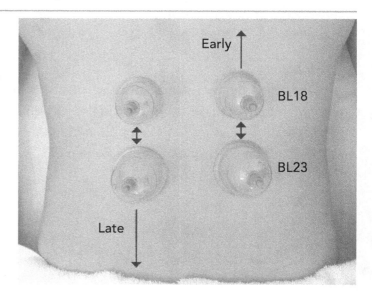

down the back if menstruation is late, and up the back one week before menstruation if menstruation tends to be early.

PAINFUL MENSTRUATION

Painful menstruation, or dysmenorrhea, tends to manifest when the period is about to start. The main symptom is lower abdominal pain or cramping; you'll also see pain in the hips, inner thighs, or lower back, and maybe also diarrhea, nausea, headache, breast tenderness, appetite changes, and mood changes. Many women who have dysmenorrhea find they do not have any underlying problems. However, common causes may include uterine fibroids, endometriosis, or pelvic inflammatory disease. Treatment for dysmenorrhea is limited.

According to TCM, stress and other emotions such as anger, worry, frustration, and anxiety strongly contribute to painful menstruation. These emotions tend to impact the Liver, the source of menstrual blood, which sends the blood to the uterus to prepare it for ovulation. A stressed Liver is a stagnant liver, with problems sending Qi and Blood to the uterus, causing pain. Cupping can be used to break up the stagnation and relieve the pain.

Another TCM cause may be cold weather or feeling cold. The Cold pathogen can enter a women's body through an opening, like the skin pores, but also the vaginal opening. Cold causes the blood vessels to constrict and restricts blood movement, which can cause pain. Cupping can help draw out the Cold pathogen, move the Blood, and stop the pain.

Overworking or having chronic illness both drain the body of Qi and Blood. Qi is needed to move Blood, so if you don't have enough Qi to move the Blood properly, the Blood can get stuck, which causes pain. Cupping can be used to move the Blood and relieve the pain.

Excessive sexual activity can also cause painful menstruation. Sexual activity uses up the Qi of the Kidneys, which are in charge of reproduction. The Kidneys are also in charge of menstruation. If they are weakened by excessive sexual activity, then they cannot control menstruation, causing pain. Cupping can help regulate the menstruation, move Qi and Blood, and relieve the pain.

CV4 *Guan Yuan—Origin Pass*

Location: The lower abdomen, on the anterior midline, three fingers' breadth (or approximately 2 inches) above the pubic bone.

When to use: For all types of painful menstruation.

Application: Use Medium to Strong Cupping for 10 to 15 minutes. Apply Moving Cupping downward toward the pubis for 3 to 5 minutes. Use every day for five days before the start of menstruation, and two days into menstruation.

Zi Gong *Child Palace*

Location: Four fingers' breadth (or approximately 3 inches) lateral to and one thumb's width (or 1 inch) below CV4.

When to use: For all types of painful menstruation.

Application: Use Medium to Strong Cupping for 10 to 15 minutes. Apply Moving Cupping downward toward the pubis for 3 to 5 minutes. Use every day for five days before the start of menstruation, and two days into menstruation.

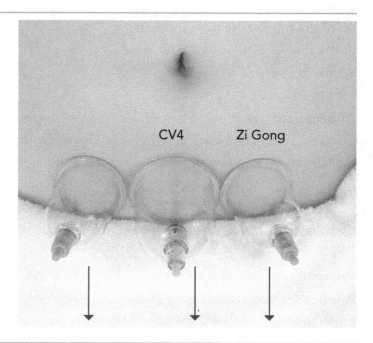

SP10 *Xue Hai–Sea of Blood*

Location: About three fingers' width (or approximately 2 inches) above the superior-medial corner of the patella.

When to use: For all types of painful menstruation.

Application: Use Medium to Strong Cupping for 10 to 15 minutes. Apply

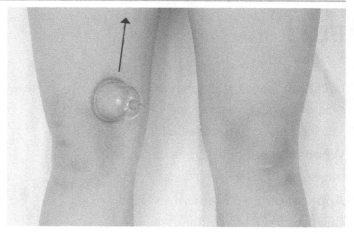

Moving Cupping up the inner thigh for 3 to 5 minutes. Use every day for five days before the start of menstruation, and two days into menstruation.

SP6 *San Yin Jiao–Three Yin Intersection*

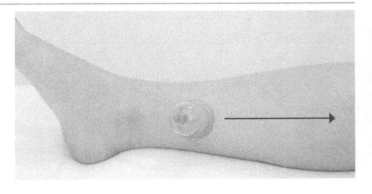

Location: Four fingers' breadth (or approximately 3 inches) above the tip of the medial malleolus, posterior to the medial border of the tibia.

When to use: For all types of painful menstruation.

Application: Use Weak, Medium, or Strong Cupping for 10 to 15 minutes. Apply Moving Cupping up the calf for 3 to 5 minutes. Use every day for five days before the start of menstruation, and two days into menstruation.

BL18 *Gan Shu–Liver Shu*

Location: 1.5 inches on either side of the spinous process of the ninth thoracic vertebra (T9).

When to use: For all types of painful menstruation.

Application: Use Medium to Strong Cupping for 10 to 15 minutes. Apply Moving Cupping down the back for 3 to 5 minutes. Use every day for five days before the start of menstruation, and two days into menstruation.

BL23 *Shen Shu–Kidney Shu*

Location: About 1.5 inches on either side of the spinous process of the second lumbar vertebra (L2).

When to use: For all types of painful menstruation.

Application: Use Medium to Strong Cupping for 10 to 15 minutes. Apply Moving Cupping down the back for 3 to 5 minutes. Use every day for five days before the start of menstruation, and two days into menstruation.

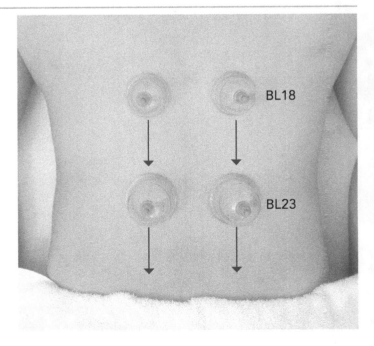

INFERTILITY

As we age, the likelihood for infertility rises. Around 50 percent of infertility is due to the female partner, and 50 percent to the male partner, but women are more likely to get tested and seek treatment than males are. This book will deal only with female infertility.

There are many causes of female infertility, one of them being hormone imbalance, which can cause a whole host of problems. Hormone imbalance can cause ovulation disorders, irregular menstruation, endometriosis, and infertility.

According to TCM, infertility can be due to a poor constitution, chronic illness, overworking, diet, and stress, which can reduce the Qi and Blood needed to sustain the embryo. Cupping can help restore your body by removing any pathogens you may have, soothe the Liver to help move Qi and Blood to the uterus, and strengthen the internal organs.

Diet also plays a big role in the body. Food is the source from which Qi and Blood are derived. If you do not eat enough or eat a lot of junk food with low nutritional value, your body will not be able to make enough Qi and Blood. Eating too much junk food can also cause a buildup of toxins in the body and harm the internal organs. Cupping can help your body's digestive system work better and remove some of the toxins from the body.

Infertility is a very complex disorder with many different causes. It is important to get an accurate diagnosis from your fertility specialist as to what is causing the infertility, so that a proper strategy can be employed. Some causes are a lot harder to fix than others are. In many cases, cupping may not be able to cure the infertility, but it can help the body work toward being healthier and thus have a better chance for pregnancy. It is also a good tool as an adjuvant treatment with other fertility treatments. Other TCM treatments such as acupuncture and herbal medicine will most likely get better results than cupping.

CV4 *Guan Yuan—Origin Pass*

Location: The lower abdomen on the anterior midline, three fingers' breadth (or approximately 2 inches) above the pubic bone.

When to use: For all types of infertility.

Application: Use Weak, Medium, to Strong Cupping for 10 to 15 minutes. Use weaker suction on someone of weaker constitution. Use stronger suction for painful menstruation.

Zi Gong *Child Palace*

Location: Four fingers' breadth (or approximately 3 inches) lateral to and one thumb's width (or approximately 1 inch) below CV4.

When to use: For all types of infertility.

Application: Use Weak, Medium, to Strong Cupping for 10 to 15 minutes. Use weaker suction for someone of a weaker constitution. Use stronger suction for painful menstruation.

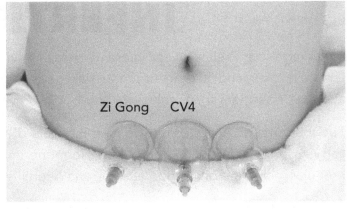

SP10 *Xue Hai–Sea of Blood*

Location: About three fingers' width (or approximately 2 inches) above the superior-medial corner of the patella.

When to use: For all types of infertility.

Application: Use Weak, Medium, to Strong Cupping for 10 to 15 minutes. Use weaker suction for someone of a weaker constitution. Use stronger suction for painful menstruation.

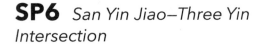

SP6 *San Yin Jiao–Three Yin Intersection*

Location: Four fingers' breadth (or approximately 3 inches) above the tip of the medial malleolus, posterior to the medial border of the tibia.

When to use: For all types of infertility.

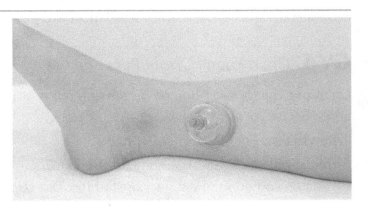

Application: Use Weak, Medium, to Strong Cupping for 10 to 15 minutes. Use weaker suction for someone of a weaker constitution. Use stronger suction for painful menstruation.

BL18 *Gan Shu–Liver Shu*

Location: 1.5 inches on either side of the spinous process of the ninth thoracic vertebra (T9).

When to use: For all types of infertility.

Application: Use Weak, Medium, to Strong Cupping for 10 to 15 minutes. Use weaker suction for someone of a weaker constitution. Use stronger suction for painful menstruation.

BL23 *Shen Shu– Kidney Shu*

Location: About 1.5 inches on either side of the spinous process of the second lumbar vertebra (L2).

When to use: For all types of infertility.

Application: Use Weak, Medium, to Strong Cupping for 10 to 15 minutes. Use weaker suction for someone of a weaker constitution. Use stronger suction for painful menstruation.

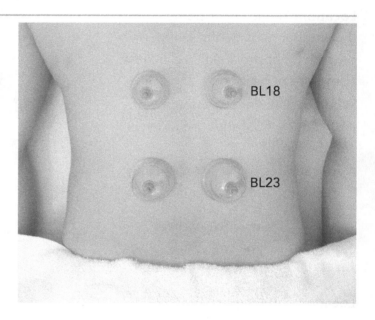

MENOPAUSAL SYNDROME

Many women suffer from perimenopausal or menopausal symptoms (such as hot flashes, night sweating, insomnia, and mood swings) months or even years before, during, and after menopause. Cupping can help to regulate the body to help with the symptoms of menopause.

According to TCM, the Kidney Essence is the basis of life. Essence is inherited from your parents when you are conceived. It starts to decline the minute you are born. Essence cannot be replenished; it can only diminish. Essence is used by the Kidneys to make two other kinds of Kidney energies: Kidney Yin and Kidney Yang. According to Yin Yang theory, women are more Yin in nature, and men are more Yang. Therefore, women require more Yin, but at the same time, they use up more of it throughout their lives. By the time they reach menopause, they've spent a lot of their Yin energy, causing them to become Yin deficient. This explains a majority of menopausal symptoms. Yin deficiency symptoms include hot flashes, night sweating, insomnia, dryness, irritability, and fatigue, to list a few. Cupping can be used to help strengthen the Kidneys, and to clear some Heat to relieve hot flashes and night sweating.

CV4 *Guan Yuan–Origin Pass*

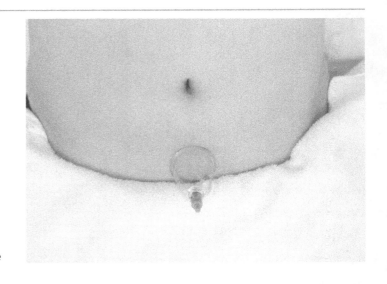

Location: The lower abdomen, on the anterior midline, three fingers' breadth (or approximately 2 inches) above the pubic bone.

When to use: For all symptoms of menopause, nourishes the Kidneys and the Yin.

Application: Use Weak to Medium Cupping for 10 to 15 minutes, twice a week.

SP6 *San Yin Jiao–Three Yin Intersection*

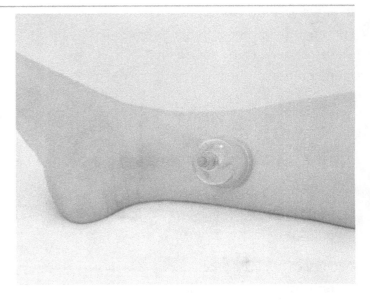

Location: Four fingers' breadth (or approximately 3 inches) above the tip of the medial malleolus, posterior to the medial border of the tibia.

When to use: For all symptoms of menopause, nourishes the Kidneys and the Yin.

Application: Use Weak to Medium Cupping for 10 to 15 minutes, twice a week.

GV14 *Da Zhui–Great Hammer*

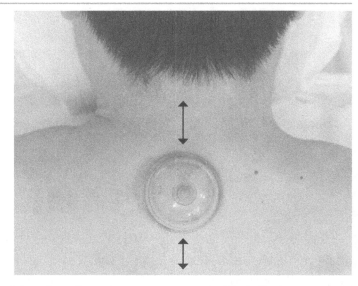

Location: Below the spinous process of the seventh cervical vertebra (C7), approximately level with the acromion (shoulders).

When to use: For night sweats and hot flashes.

Application: Use Medium to Strong Cupping for 10 to 15 minutes, twice a week. Apply Moving Cupping up and down the neck to clear Heat to treat hot flashes and night sweats. Use Bleeding Cupping once a week if hot flashes and night sweats are severe.

BL15 *Xin Shu–Heart Shu*

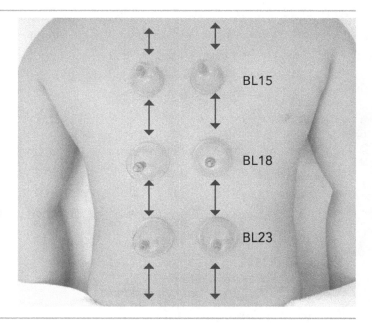

Location: 1.5 inches on either side of the spinous process of the fifth thoracic vertebra (T5).

When to use: For insomnia, irritability, short temper, restlessness, hot flashes, night sweats.

Application: Use Weak to Medium Cupping for 10 –to 15 minutes, twice a week. Use Moving Cupping up and down the back for hot flashes, night sweats, irritability, restlessness, and short temper.

BL18 *Gan Shu–Liver Shu*

Location: 1.5 inches on either side of the spinous process of the ninth thoracic vertebra (T9).

When to use: For depression, irritability, short temper, restlessness.

Application: Use Weak to Medium Cupping for 10 to 15 minutes, twice a week. Use Moving Cupping up and down the back for irritability, restlessness, and short temper.

BL23 *Shen Shu–Kidney Shu*

Location: About 1.5 inches on either side of the spinous process of the second lumbar vertebra (L2).

When to use: For all symptoms of menopause and nourishing the Kidneys.

Application: Use Weak to Medium Cupping for 10 to 15 minutes, twice a week.

COMMON COLD

Generally harmless and self-limiting, a common cold will typically resolve on its own. However, if left untreated, it can cause secondary infections like ear infections, strep throat, pneumonia, or bronchiolitis.

According to TCM, common colds are due to pathogenic Wind attacking the superficial layers of your body, as well as a weak or unprepared immune system. Wind can also bring other pathogens with it, like Cold, Heat, Dampness, or Dryness. These pathogens determine what types of symptoms you may experience with your cold. Cold pathogen causes strong chills, a runny nose, and strong body aches. Heat pathogen causes a sore throat, a hacking cough, and fever. Dampness pathogen causes body aches, congestion, and lots of phlegm. Dryness pathogen causes a dry sore throat and dry cough.

If your immune system is even temporarily down, like when you don't get enough sleep, don't dress warmly, or are in cold weather, Wind can penetrate your immune system, bringing the other pathogens with it. The best way to get rid of the Wind in TCM is to open the pores and kick the Wind back out. Cupping is an excellent way to do this.

Treatment *Common Cold*

Location: Entire chest (avoid the nipples).

When to use: For any type of common cold, especially if there is cough, chest congestion, nasal congestion, wheezing, or shortness of breath.

Application: Use Moving Cupping with weak to medium suction across the chest to clear out the pathogen from the lungs. Start from the middle and move outward, and from top to bottom, avoiding going over the nipples.

GV14 *Da Zhui–Great Hammer*

Location: Below the spinous process of the seventh cervical vertebra (C7), approximately level with the acromion (shoulders).

When to use: For any type of common cold, but especially good for sore throat and fever.

Application: Use Medium to Strong Cupping for 10 to 15 minutes, once a day, until cold is gone. Apply Moving Cupping up and down the neck to clear Heat for fever and sore throat. Use Bleeding Cupping if there is high fever.

BL12 *Feng Men–Wind Gate*

Location: About 1.5 inches on either side of the spinous process of the second thoracic vertebra (T2).

When to use: For any type of common cold.

Application: Use Moving Cupping with medium to strong suction up and down the back for 10 to 15 minutes, once a day, until cold is gone.

BL13 *Fei Shu–Lung Shu*

Location: About 1.5 inches on either side of the spinous process of the third thoracic vertebra (T3).

When to use: Used for any type of common cold.

Application: Use Moving Cupping with medium to strong suction up and down the back for 10 to 15 minutes, once a day, until cold is gone.

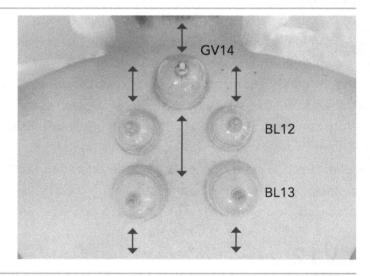

ST36 *Zu San Li–Leg Three Miles*

Location: Four fingers' width below the inferior-lateral corner of the patella, and one thumb's width (or about 1 inch) lateral to the tibia (shinbone).

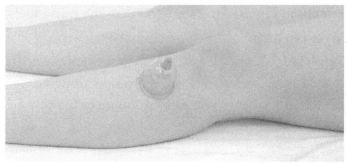

When to use: For a cold that drags on for a long time, or frequent sickness.

Application: Use Weak to Medium Cupping for 10 to 15 minutes, once a day, until cold is gone.

STOMACH FLU

In medicine, there is no treatment for the stomach flu, or viral gastroenteritis. The best treatment is getting enough rest and staying hydrated. The stomach flu is self-limiting and generally passes after a few days. Prevent it by avoiding food or water that is suspect to contamination, washing your hands frequently, and avoiding people who have it. If you do get it, it is better to avoid certain foods until you feel better, then slowly reintroduce them.

In TCM, the stomach flu is due to an external pathogen, usually Dampness, combined with either Cold or Heat. The Dampness gets into the body by hitching a ride with the Wind pathogen. The Dampness likes to attack the Spleen. The Spleen doesn't like to be damp, as it is the Spleen's job to get rid of pathogenic water or liquid wastes from the body. The Spleen is also in charge of the digestive system, and when it gets attacked by Dampness, it cannot control the bowels properly nor get rid of pathogenic water. The stools become very watery, leading to diarrhea. When Dampness invades the Stomach, you will fee very full and bloated, as if you just drank a lot of water. Dampness also prevents the Stomach from sending food down to the Small Intestines. The food has to go somewhere, but since it cannot go down, it will go back up, leading to nausea and vomiting. Body aches and fever are due to the Wind pathogen attacking the body. Cupping can help suck out the pathogenic Wind and Dampness from the body. It can also help to harmonize the Spleen, Stomach, and Small Intestines, helping you recover quicker.

CV12 *Zhong Wan—Central Stomach*

Location: On the anterior midline of the body, halfway between the sternum and umbilicus.

When to use: For any type stomach flu, especially if there is nausea or vomiting.

Application: Use Weak to Medium Cupping for 10 to 15 minutes. Apply Moving Cupping in a counterclockwise direction to slow down bowel movement and stop diarrhea, or downward to stop nausea and vomiting. Do some Flash Cupping to clear the pathogen.

CV6 *Qi Hai—Sea of Qi*

Location: On the anterior midline of the body, one thumb's length (or around 1.5 inches) below the umbilicus.

When to use: To strengthen the body, especially if there is diarrhea.

Application: Use Weak to Medium Cupping for 10 to 15 minutes, applying Moving Cupping in a counterclockwise direction to slow down bowel movement and stop diarrhea.

ST25 *Tian Shu—Celestial Pivot*

Location: Around three fingers' breadth (or approximately 2 inches) on either side of the umbilicus.

When to use: To stop diarrhea.

Application: Use Weak to Medium Cupping for 10 to 15 minutes, applying Moving Cupping in a counterclockwise direction to slow down bowel movement and stop diarrhea.

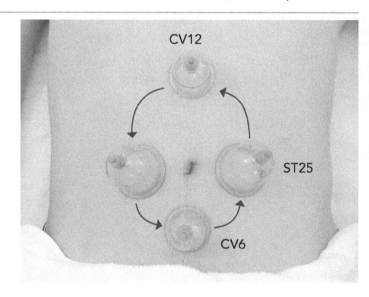

BL20 *Pi Shu—Spleen Shu*

Location: 1.5 inches on either side of the spinous process of the eleventh thoracic vertebra (T11).

When to use: To clear pathogen from the digestive system, and to stop vomiting and diarrhea

Application: Do Weak to Medium Cupping for 10 to 15 minutes, applying Moving Cupping up the back to slow down bowel movement and stop diarrhea, and down the back to stop nausea and vomiting. Do some Flash Cupping to clear the pathogen.

BL25 *Da Chang Shu– Large Intestine Shu*

Location: 1.5 inches on either side of the spinous process of the fourth lumbar vertebra (L4).

When to use: For any type of large intestine problem. Helps to stop diarrhea.

Application: Use Weak to Medium Cupping for 10 to 15 minutes, applying Moving Cupping up the back to slow down bowel movement and stop diarrhea. Do some Flash Cupping to clear the pathogen.

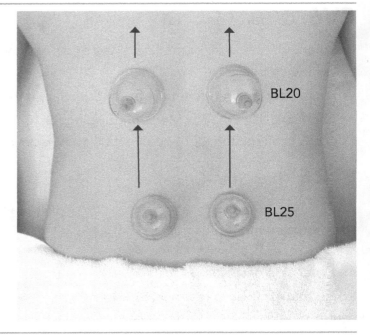

ST36 *Zu San Li–Leg Three Miles*

Location: Four fingers' width (or approximately 3 inches) below the inferior-lateral corner of the patella, about 1 inch lateral to the tibia (shinbone).

When to use: To help improve the digestive system as a whole, and to help stop diarrhea and vomiting.

Application: Use Flash Cupping with medium suction for 10 to 15 minutes to get rid of the pathogen.

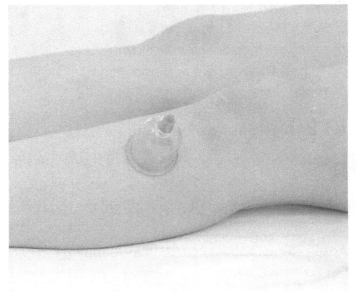

ALLERGIES

There are many types of allergies, but the most common are allergies to dust, pets, medication, food, and air pollution, as well as seasonal allergies. Those that are caused from inhaling substances, such as seasonal allergies, usually have similar respiratory symptoms, such as runny nose, stuffy nose, sneezing, wheezing, shortness of breath, cough, headache, feverish sensation, fatigue, and rashes. Allergies that involve ingestion, such as food allergies, mostly have digestive symptoms, such as swelling of the lips, tongue, or throat; abdominal pain; nausea, vomiting, or diarrhea; fatigue; or skin rash.

According to TCM, allergies are due to a weakened immune system, which we call Wei Qi, or Defensive Qi. Defensive Qi is made by and distributed throughout the body by the Lungs. If the Lungs are weak, they cannot make enough Wei Qi to protect against pathogens, which then mainly attack the Lungs. Cupping is a good way to suck the pathogen out of the body, reducing the allergic response. The Lungs also control the skin, so some people may get skin rashes or hives. Food allergies are usually due to a deficiency of the Spleen, which controls the digestive system. Cupping can help strengthen the Lungs and the Spleen, which can help prevent allergic reactions.

Treatment *Allergies*

Location: Entire chest (avoid the nipples).

When to use: For seasonal allergies, especially if there is cough, chest congestion, nasal congestion, wheezing, or shortness of breath.

Application: Use Moving Cupping with low to medium suction across the chest for 1 to 2 minutes every other day to clear allergens from the Lungs. Start from the middle and move outward and from top to bottom, avoiding going over the nipples.

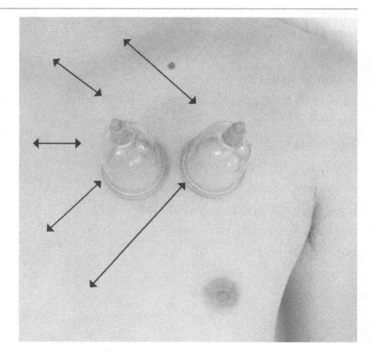

GV14 *Da Zhui–Great Hammer*

Location: Below the spinous process of the seventh cervical vertebra (C7), approximately level with the acromion (shoulders).

When to use: For all types of allergies, especially seasonal allergies.

Application: To clear inflammation, use Moving Cupping with medium to strong suction up and down the neck for 10 to 15 minutes, every other day, during allergy season. Use Flash Cupping for 1 minute to clear pathogens.

BL12 *Feng Men–Wind Gate*

Location: About 1.5 inches on either side of the spinous process of the second thoracic vertebra (T2).

When to use: For most allergies, especially seasonal allergies and skin reactions.

Application: Use Medium to Strong Cupping for 10 to 15 minutes, every other day, during allergy season. Use Moving Cupping up and down the back for 1 minute to remove pathogens and relieve allergy symptoms.

BL13 *Fei Shu–Lung Shu*

Location: About 1.5 inches on either side of the spinous process of the third thoracic vertebra (T3).

When to use: For most allergies, especially seasonal allergies and skin reactions.

Application: Use Medium to Strong Cupping for 10 to 15 minutes every other day during allergy season. Use Moving Cupping up and down the back for 1 minute to remove pathogens and relieve allergy symptoms.

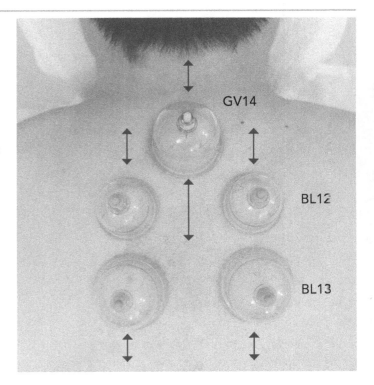

BL20 *Pi Shu–Spleen Shu*

Location: 1.5 inches on either side of the spinous process of the eleventh thoracic vertebra (T11).

When to use: For mild food allergies and food intolerances.

Application: Use Medium to Strong Cupping for 10 to 15 minutes immediately after experiencing symptoms. Use Moving Cupping up and down the back for 1 minute to remove pathogen and relieve allergy symptoms. Do Flash Cupping for 1 minute to remove pathogen.

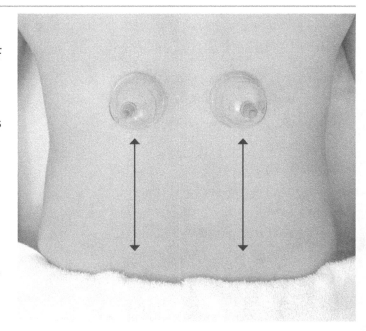

ST36 *Zu San Li–Leg Three Miles*

Location: Four fingers' width (or approximately 3 inches) below the inferior-lateral corner of the patella, and one thumb's width (or about 1 inch) lateral to the tibia (shinbone).

When to use: For strengthening the immune system as a whole. Used mainly for prevention during allergy season. Also good for food allergies as it can strengthen digestive system.

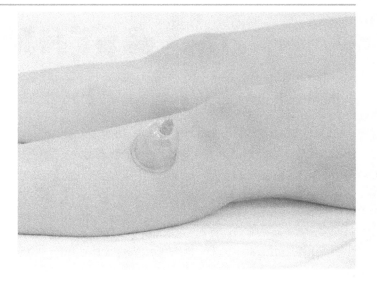

Application: Use Weak to Medium Cupping for 10 to 15 minutes, two to three times a week prior to or during allergy season. Can also use when experiencing food allergies.

BL40 *Wei Zhong– Bend Middle*

Location: Middle of the popliteal crease (crease behind the knees).

When to use: For allergies that cause skin conditions such as hives, eczema, or itchiness.

Application: Use Weak to Medium Cupping for 10 to 15 minutes, immediately after getting symptoms. Use Flash Cupping for 1 minute or Bleeding Cupping if skin condition is intense or acute.

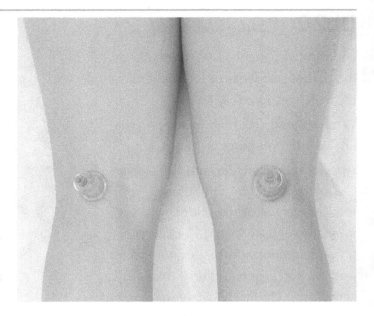

ASTHMA

Asthma is an inflammatory disease that causes the airways in the lungs to swell and produce extra mucus, narrowing the airways and causing difficulty breathing.

According to TCM, asthma is due to the Lungs' inability to allow Qi or air to descend into the body. Instead, Qi backs up, which causes coughing, wheezing, and shortness of breath. The Lungs are also in charge of descending water to the Kidneys, but if Qi cannot descend, water cannot either. Therefore, water accumulates in the Lungs, causing mucus to build up.

There are a few reasons why the Lungs cannot descend their Qi. If the asthma is due to allergies, then external pathogens have entered the Lungs, blocking Qi's descent. Additionally, lungs weakened by not enough exercise, crying too much, overexertion, illness, premature birth, or an inborn condition become too weak to work and cannot descend their own Qi, causing asthma. Cupping can help suck out the external pathogens, strengthen the Lungs, and help the Lung descend Qi.

If the asthma is diet related, then it is due to a weak Spleen unable to digest the food, leading Dampness and Phlegm to build up. The Phlegm makes it way to the Lungs, blocking the Lung Qi from descending. Cupping can help strengthen the Spleen, remove some of the Dampness and Phlegm, and descend Lung Qi.

If the asthma is triggered by anxiety or stress, the Liver cannot move Qi throughout the whole body. Cupping can help relax the Liver, move Qi, and descend the Lung Qi. Asthma can also be due to weak Kidneys, which are said to help the Lungs descend the Qi by grasping the Qi downward. However, if the Kidneys are weakened, it cannot grasp the Lung Qi, which will float back up, causing asthma. Cupping can help strengthen the Kidneys and help the Lung Qi descend.

Treatment *Asthma*

Location: Sternum.

When to use: To clear asthma of any type; for cough, chest congestion, wheezing, or shortness of breath.

Application: Use Moving Cupping down the sternum starting just under the throat and ending at the stomach for 1 to 2 minutes every other day.

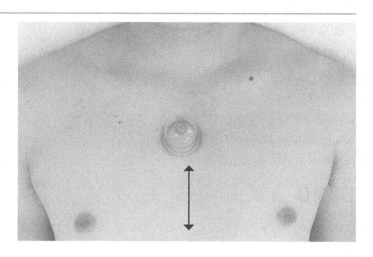

GV14 *Da Zhui—Great Hammer*

Location: Below the spinous process of the seventh cervical vertebra (C7), approximately level with the acromion (shoulders).

When to use: For all types of asthma.

Application: Use Medium to Strong Cupping for 10 to 15 minutes every other day during asthma episodes. Use Moving Cupping down the middle of the back to stop asthma, and Flash Cupping if asthma is due to allergies.

BL12 *Feng Men—Wind Gate*

Location: About 1.5 inches on either side of the spinous process of the second thoracic vertebra (T2).

When to use: For all types of asthma, especially asthma due to allergies.

Application: Use Medium to Strong Cupping for 10 to 15 minutes every other day during an asthma episode. Use Moving Cupping down the back for 1 minute to stop asthma and remove pathogens or allergens.

BL13 *Fei Shu–Lung Shu*

Location: About 1.5 inches on either side of the spinous process of the third thoracic vertebra (T3).

When to use: For all types of asthma, especially asthma due to allergies.

Application: Use Medium to Strong Cupping for 10 to 15 minutes every other day during an asthma episode. Use Moving Cupping down the back for 1 minute to stop asthma and remove pathogens or allergens.

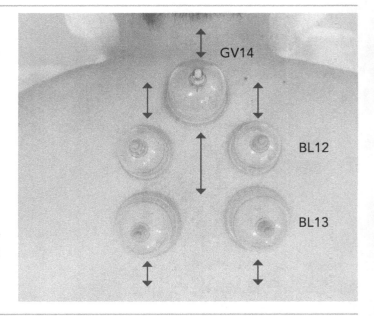

BL20 *Pi Shu–Spleen Shu*

Location: 1.5 inches on either side of the spinous process of the eleventh thoracic vertebra (T11).

When to use: For diet-related asthma.

Application: Use Medium to Strong Cupping for 10 to 15 minutes immediately after symptoms start. Use Moving Cupping down the back for 1e minute to stop asthma and remove pathogens or allergens.

BL23 *Shen Shu–Kidney Shu*

Location: About 1.5 inches on either side of the spinous process of the second lumbar vertebra (L2).

When to use: For chronic asthma.

Application: Use Weak or Medium Cupping for 10 to 15 minutes, twice a week, together with BL13.

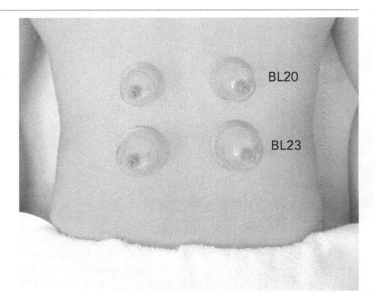

ACNE

According to TCM, acne is due to excess Heat and Dampness in the body. Heat manifests as rashes, pimples, redness, and other skin inflammation. Toxins (chemicals in soaps, shampoos, or makeup) can cause Heat to build up in the skin. Greasy, spicy, deep-fried, barbecued, or baked foods, as well as drinks such as coffee, alcohol, or sodas also tend to create Heat.

In TCM, we split hormonal activities into Yin and Yang. Yang hormones testosterone, cortisol, or thyroxin tend to make you more active, energetic, and hot. Yin hormones tend to make people more relaxed and less active, and preserve the body more. An excess of Yang hormones will generate Heat in the body. Cupping can help balance the Yin and Yang in the body.

Bacteria thrive in Dampness, which happens when the Spleen cannot transform and transport body fluids. Dampness manifests as oily skin, swelling, cysts, pimples, pus, or fluid discharge. It can be due to excessive consumption of greasy, cold, or raw foods, irregular eating habits, living in a damp environment, or working too hard. Cupping can help with acne by clearing Heat and draining Dampness from the body.

GV14 *Da Zhui–Great Hammer*

Location: Below the spinous process of the seventh cervical vertebra (C7), approximately level with the acromion (shoulders).

When to use: For all types of acne, especially if it is red or inflamed.

Application: Use Medium to Strong Cupping for 10 to 15 minutes, twice a week if chronic, and every other day for sporadic acne. Use Moving Cupping up and down the neck for 1 minute to clear heat and inflammation, Flash Cupping for 1 minute to clear more Heat, and Bleeding Cupping for extreme cases.

BL12 *Feng Men–Wind Gate*

Location: About 1.5 inches on either side of the spinous process of the second thoracic vertebra (T2).

When to use: For all kinds of skin conditions, especially those due to weather or the environment.

Application: Use Medium to Strong Cupping for 10 to 15 minutes, twice a week if chronic, and every other day for sporadic acne. Use Moving Cupping up and down the back for 1 minute to remove the pathogen and relieve symptoms.

BL13 *Fei Shu–Lung Shu*

Location: About 1.5 inches on either side of the spinous process of the third thoracic vertebra (T3).

When to use: For all kinds of skin conditions, especially those due to weather or the environment.

Application: Use Medium to Strong Cupping for 10 to 15 minutes, twice a week if chronic, every other day for sporadic acne. Use Moving Cupping up and down the back for 1 minute to remove the pathogen and relieve symptoms.

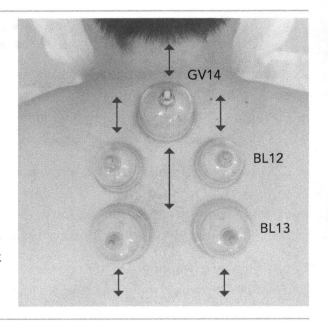

BL17 *Ge Shu–Diaphragm Shu*

Location: 1.5 inches on either side of the spinous process of the seventh thoracic vertebra (T7).

When to use: For acne that is red, inflamed, or itchy.

Application: Use Medium to Strong Cupping for 10 to 15 minutes, twice a week if chronic, and every other day for sporadic acne. Use Moving Cupping up and down the back for 1 minute to remove the pathogen and relieve symptoms.

BL20 *Pi Shu–Spleen Shu*

Location: 1.5 inches on either side of the spinous process of the eleventh thoracic vertebra (T11).

When to use: For whiteheads or acne that is food related or pus filled.

Application: Use Medium to Strong Cupping for 10 to 15 minutes, twice a week if chronic, and every other day for sporadic acne. Use Moving Cupping up and down the back for 1 minute to remove the pathogen and relieve symptoms.

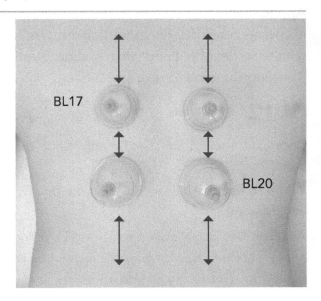

BL40 *Wei Zhong–Bend Middle*

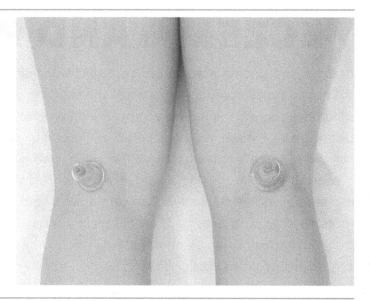

Location: Middle of the popliteal crease (crease behind the knees).

When to use: For all skin conditions, especially if red, inflamed, or itchy.

Application: Use Weak to Medium Cupping for 10 to 15 minutes immediately after getting symptoms. Can also use Flash Cupping for 1 minute or Bleeding Cupping if skin condition is intense or acute.

SP10 *Xue Hai–Sea of Blood*

Location: About three fingers' width (or approximately 2 inches) above the superior-medial corner of the patella.

When to use: For all skin conditions, especially if red, inflamed, or itchy.

Application: Use Weak to Medium Cupping for 10 to 15 minutes immediately after getting symptoms. Can also use Flash Cupping for 1 minute if skin condition is intense or acute.

SP9 *Yin Ling Quan–Yin Mound Spring*

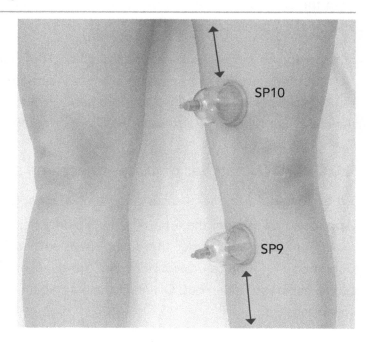

Location: In the depression just below and behind the medial condyle of the tibia.

When to use: For whiteheads or acne that is food related or pus filled.

Application: Use Weak to Medium Cupping for 10 to 15 minutes immediately after getting symptoms. Can also use Moving Cupping up and down the leg for 1 minute if skin condition is intense or acute.

ECZEMA AND PSORIASIS

Eczema and psoriasis are often confused with each other. They may look similar at first sight, and some doctors who are not specialists in dermatology may not be able to tell the difference. Eczema is a chronic skin condition due to a hypersensitivity of the skin. It can be triggered by coming into contact with certain substances like dyes, fabrics, or soaps. It can cause quite intense itching. When you scratch it, it may bleed and ooze. Psoriasis is a chronic and recurrent skin disorder characterized by thickened skin that looks like slightly elevated silvery-white scales. The skin underneath the scales is usually inflamed and red, more so than with eczema. The cause of psoriasis is unknown, but there seems to be a genetic predisposition. Neither eczema nor psoriasis can be cured, but they can be treated similarly using ointments and creams.

According to TCM, both eczema and psoriasis are treated similarly, as they are both usually caused by pathogenic Wind, Dampness, or Heat attacking the skin. Wind likes to attack the outer regions of the body and can bring with it the Dampness pathogen. When you scratch your skin and it oozes, this is the Dampness seeping out. Wind can also bring the Heat pathogen, making the skin red and inflamed. Dampness and Heat can also come from inside the body, mostly through fried, greasy, or spicy foods; coffee; alcohol; and dairy. If these toxins cannot be eliminated, they get trapped in the body and must come out, sometimes from the skin as eczema and psoriasis. Cupping can help to extract the Wind, Dampness, and Heat from the body.

Eczema and psoriasis can also come from Blood deficiency. When Blood is deficient, it cannot send nutrients to the skin, causing skin to become malnourished, dry, and cracked. Blood deficiency can also cause Wind to more easily invade the empty blood vessels, which causes itchiness. Cupping can help clear the Wind, bringing fresh Blood and nutrients to the area.

Location *Patches of skin with eczema and psoriasis*

When to use: For general cases of eczema and psoriasis.

Application: Disinfect the area with the eczema or psoriasis with 70 percent alcohol, use a lancet to prick a few holes there, and use Bleeding Cupping with weak suction that is only strong enough to draw blood from the skin. Leave cup on for about 1 minute after the blood has been drawn out. Disinfect the area again, then bandage it. Can be done once a week per area.

GV14 *Da Zhui–Great Hammer*

Location: Below the spinous process of the seventh cervical vertebra (C7), approximately level with the acromion (shoulders).

When to use: For all types of eczema or psoriasis, especially if it is red or inflamed, or due to allergies.

Application: Use Medium to Strong Cupping for 10 to 15 minutes, twice a week if chronic or every other day if the lesions are just starting to come out. Use Moving Cupping up and down the neck for 1 minute to clear Heat and inflammation. Use Flash Cupping for 1 minute to clear more Heat. For extreme cases, use Bleeding Cupping.

BL12 *Feng Men–Wind Gate*

Location: About 1.5 inches on either side of the spinous process of the second thoracic vertebra (T2).

When to use: For all kinds of skin conditions, especially those due to allergies, weather, or the environment.

Application: Use Medium to Strong Cupping for 10 to 15 minutes, twice a week if chronic, or every other day if the lesions are just starting to come out. Use Moving Cupping up and down the back for 1 minute to remove the pathogen and relieve symptoms.

BL13 *Fei Shu–Lung Shu*

Location: About 1.5 inches on either side of the spinous process of the third thoracic vertebra (T3).

When to use: For all kinds of skin conditions, especially those due to allergies, the weather, or the environment.

Application: Use Medium to Strong Cupping for 10 to 15 minutes, twice a week if chronic, or every other day if the lesions are just starting

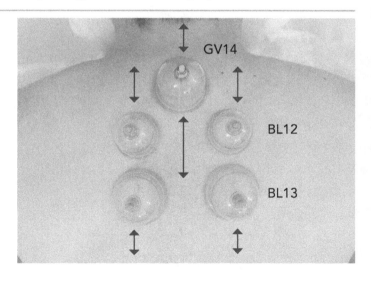

to come out. Use Moving Cupping up and down the back for 1 minute to remove the pathogen and relieve symptoms.

BL17 *Ge Shu–Diaphragm Shu*

Location: 1.5 inches on either side of the spinous process of the seventh thoracic vertebra (T7).

When to use: For eczema or psoriasis that is red, inflamed, or itchy.

Application: Use Medium to Strong Cupping for 10 to 15 minutes, twice a week if chronic, or every other day if the lesions are just starting to come out. Use Moving Cupping up and down the back for 1 minute to remove the pathogen and relieve symptoms.

BL20 *Pi Shu–Spleen Shu*

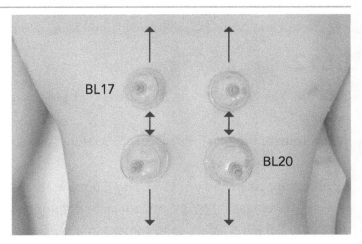

Location: 1.5 inches on either side of the spinous process of the eleventh thoracic vertebra (T11).

When to use: For eczema or psoriasis that is food related.

Application: Use Medium to Strong Cupping for 10 to 15 minutes, twice a week if chronic, or every other day if the lesions are just starting to come out. Use Moving Cupping up and down the back for 1 minute to remove the pathogen and relieve symptoms.

BL40 *Wei Zhong–Bend Middle*

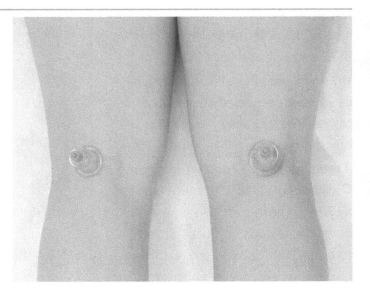

Location: Middle of the popliteal crease (crease behind the knees).

When to use: For all skin conditions, especially if red, inflamed, or itchy.

Application: Use Weak to Medium Cupping for 10 to 15 minutes immediately after getting symptoms. Can also use Flash Cupping for 1 minute or Bleeding Cupping if skin condition is intense or acute.

SP10 *Xue Hai—Sea of Blood*

Location: About three fingers' width (or approximately 2 inches) above the superior-medial corner of the patella.

When to use: Used for all skin conditions, especially if red, inflamed, or itchy.

Application: Use Weak to Medium Cupping for 10 to 15 minutes immediately after getting symptoms. Can also use Flash Cupping for 1 minute if skin condition is intense or acute.

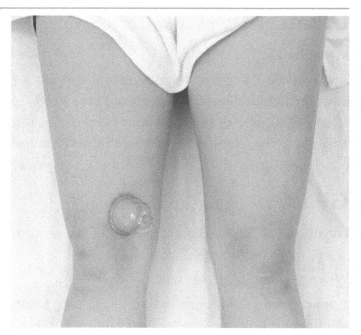

SHINGLES

Also called herpes zoster, shingles is due to an infection by the varicella-zoster virus, the same virus that causes chickenpox. However, unlike most infections that go away, the varicella-zoster virus hides in the nerve cells for years or even decades before reemerging. When it reemerges, it is called shingles. Symptoms of shingles are painful red skin rashes that are localized in a band or stripe on only one side of the body. Its distribution depends on the area of the body controlled by the nerve the virus was hiding in, and it only attacks those regions. Other symptoms are fever, chills, fatigue, and muscle weakness. Shingles are usually triggered by poor immune system. It usually goes away by itself after a few weeks, goes back to hiding, and does not return.

According to TCM, shingles is also due to the external pathogens Wind and extreme Heat attacking the skin. The Heat toxin builds up in the skin, causing painful red rashes. Wind causes the skin to feel itchy. In TCM, pathogens can also lay latent in the body, popping up years later. In the case of shingles, it tends to come out in the Liver channel, which flows through the sides of the body, where shingles is commonly found. The Liver belongs to the Wood element, which is the perfect fuel for Heat and Fire. Cupping can help clear out the pathogens, reduce inflammation, and stop the pain.

Location *Patches of skin with shingles*

When to use: For shingles.

Application: Disinfect the area with the shingles with 70 percent alcohol, use a lancet to prick the papules in the area, and use Bleeding Cupping with weak suction that is only strong enough to draw blood from the skin. Leave cup on for around one minute, or long enough to draw a few drops of blood from each hole. Disinfect the area again and bandage. Can be done once every two to three days during the shingles episode.

GV14 *Da Zhui—Great Hammer*

Location: Below the spinous process of the seventh cervical vertebra (C7), approximate y level with the acromion (shoulders).

When to use: For shingles.

Application: Use Medium to Strong Cupping for 10 to 15 minutes every other day during the shingles episode. Use Moving Cupping up and down the neck for 1 minute to clear Heat and inflammation. Use Flash Cupping for 1 minute to clear more Heat. For extreme cases, use Bleeding Cupping.

BL12 *Feng Men—Wind Gate*

Location: About 1.5 inches on either side of the spinous process of the second thoracic vertebra (T2).

When to use: For all kinds of skin conditions, including shingles.

Application: Medium to Strong Cupping for 10-15 minutes, use every other day during the shingles episode. Can use Moving Cupping up and down the neck for one minute to clear Heat and inflammation. Can use Flash Cupping for one minute to clear more Heat.

BL13 *Fei Shu—Lung Shu*

Location: about 1.5 inch on either side of the spinous process of the third thoracic vertebra (T3).

When to use: For all kinds of skin conditions, including shingles.

Application: Use Medium to Strong Cupping for 10 to 15 minutes every other day during the shingles

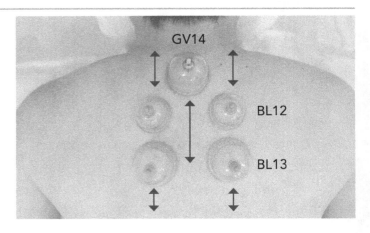

episode. Use Moving Cupping up and down the neck for 1 minute to clear Heat and inflammation. Can use Flash Cupping for 1 minute to clear more Heat.

BL17 *Ge Shu–Diaphragm Shu*

Location: 1.5 inches on either side of the spinous process of the seventh thoracic vertebra (T7).

When to use: For all kinds of skin conditions, including shingles.

Application: Use Medium to Strong Cupping for 10 to 15 minutes every other day during the shingles episode. Use Moving Cupping up and down the neck for 1 minute to clear Heat and inflammation. Use Flash Cupping for 1 minute to clear more Heat.

BL19 *Dan Shu–Gallbladder Shu*

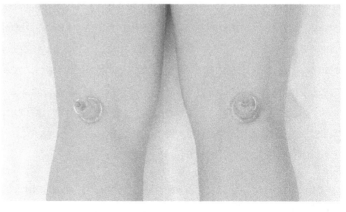

Location: 1.5 inches on either side of the spinous process of the tenth thoracic vertebra (T10).

When to use: For shingles.

Application: Use Medium to Strong Cupping for 10 to 15 minutes every other day during the shingles episode. Use Moving Cupping up and down the neck for 1 minute to clear Heat and inflammation. Use Flash Cupping for 1 minute to clear more Heat.

BL40 *Wei Zhong–Bend Middle*

Location: Middle of the popliteal crease (crease behind the knees).

When to use: For all skin conditions, including shingles.

Application: Use Medium Cupping for 10 to 15 minutes every other day during shingles episode. Can also use Flash Cupping for 1 minute or Bleeding Cupping if skin condition is intense or acute.

SP10 *Xue Hai—Sea of Blood*

Location: Three fingers' width (or approximately 2 inches) medial and superior to the superior-medial corner of the patella.

When to use: For all skin conditions, including shingles.

Application: Use Medium Cupping for 10 to 15 minutes every other day during shingles episode. Can also use Flash Cupping for 1 minute if skin condition is intense or acute.

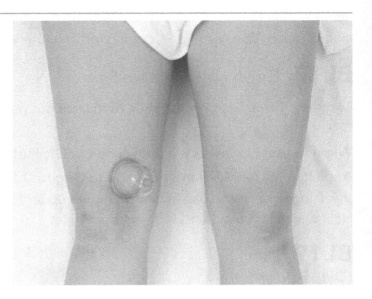

ANXIETY AND STRESS

Everyone experiences anxiety or stress in their life. Its frequency can depend on your home environment, school or work environment, relationships, and personality. Usually, once a stressful situation passes, the anxiety or stress will pass as well. However, in some people, anxiety can be so bad that they are anxious or stressed even after the situation has passed. It can prevent them from living a normal life, in which case it can become an anxiety disorder.

There are different types of anxiety disorders. Panic disorders are similar to anxiety except they hit very hard and suddenly. Symptoms can include palpitations, sweating, light-headedness, headache, nausea, shortness of breath, and hyperventilation. Social anxiety disorder is anxiety specifically in social interactions, where you may feel embarrassed or self-conscious, as if others are judging you. This can cause palpitations, sweating, and trouble focusing. Generalized anxiety disorder is having excessive and unrealistic or exaggerated worry about trivial things, or things you have no control over. Symptoms can include general muscle tension, restlessness, irritability, headaches, fatigue, nausea, frequent urination, insomnia, teeth grinding, or poor appetite.

According to TCM, the emotions are closely linked with the internal organs, so not only can anxiety and stress cause health problems, but health problems themselves can cause a person to feel anxious or stressed. The Heart and Liver are said to be the two organs that control all emotions in the body. At the same time, emotions can harm these two organs more so than your other organs, especially anxiety and stress. The Liver is responsible for moving Qi throughout the body, and the Heart is responsible for moving Blood throughout the body. If they both are hampered by anxiety and stress, Qi and Blood won't be able to move freely through the body, causing many problems, including muscle tension, headaches, and fatigue. Cupping can help move Qi and Blood throughout the body, helping to relieve these symptoms. Since the Liver and Heart control all emotions, when they get affected by anxiety and stress, other emotions also get worse, such as depression, restlessness, short-temperedness, irritability, and insomnia. Cupping is very relaxing and can help to release some of the built-up tension and emotions.

When the Liver is under stress, it cannot help the Spleen with digestion, which in turn causes poor appetite, poor digestion, and sometimes stress eating. The emotion associated with the Spleen is overthinking, and anxiety is a form of overthinking, which can also weaken the Spleen and your entire digestive system. Cupping can be used to strengthen the digestive system and harmonize the Liver and the Spleen.

If your Liver, Heart, or Spleen is weakened from illness, lack of sleep, or overworking, this can lead your body to be more prone to anxiety and stress, and less able to deal with these emotions. Cupping can help you to strengthen these organs, and help your body be able to deal with these emotions.

GB20 *Feng Chi–Wind Pool*

Location: In the depression between the sternocleidomastoid muscle and the trapezius muscle, just at the base of the skull.

When to use: For neck and shoulder tension due to anxiety or stress.

Application: GB20 is actually within the hairline, so a cup cannot be placed directly on it, but you can place it as close to the hairline as possible. Use Weak or Medium Cupping twice a week for 10 to 15 minutes. Use stronger suction if there is more tension, and weaker suction for relaxation.

GB21 *Jian Jing–Shoulder Well*

Location: On the most superior part of the shoulder, directly above the nipple, or halfway from the spine to the deltoid muscle.

When to use: For neck and shoulder tension due to anxiety or stress.

Application: Use Weak or Medium Cupping twice a week for 10 to 15 minutes. Use stronger suction if there is more tension, and weaker suction for relaxation.

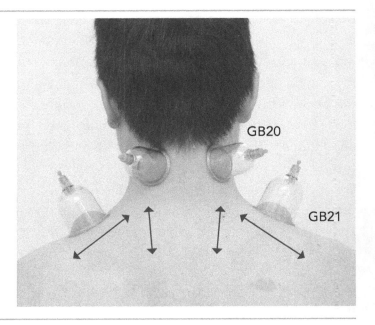

BL15 *Xin Shu–Heart Shu*

Location: 1.5 inches on either side of the spinous process of the fifth thoracic vertebra (T5).

When to use: For any mental symptoms, including anxiety, stress, insomnia, irritability, shorttemperedness, or restlessness.

Application: Use Weak to Medium Cupping for 10 to 15 minutes, twice a week. Use less suction for a gentle and relaxing treatment, and slightly stronger suction if there is muscle tension in the area.

BL18 *Gan Shu–Liver Shu*

Location: 1.5 inches on either side of the spinous process of the ninth thoracic vertebra (T9).

When to use: For any mental symptoms, including anxiety, stress, insomnia, irritability, short-temperedness, restlessness, or depression.

Application: Use Weak to Medium Cupping for 10 to 15 minutes, twice a week. Use less suction for a gentle and relaxing treatment. Use slightly stronger suction or Moving Cupping up and down the back for general muscle tension.

BL20 *Pi Shu–Spleen Shu*

Location: 1.5 inches on either side of the spinous process of the eleventh thoracic vertebra (T11).

When to use: For overthinking and anxiety, especially if it affects digestion, such as nausea, vomiting, indigestion, diarrhea, constipation, bloating, etc.

Application: Use Weak to Medium Cupping for 10 to 15 minutes, twice a week. Use less suction for a gentle and relaxing treatment.

BL23 *Shen Shu–Kidney Shu*

Location: About 1.5 inches on either side of the spinous process of the second lumbar vertebra (L2).

When to use: For anxiety or stress due to fear and phobias, especially when frequent urination, fatigue, or sexual dysfunction is involved.

Application: Use Weak to Medium Cupping for 10 to 15 minutes, twice a week. Use less suction for a gentle and relaxing treatment.

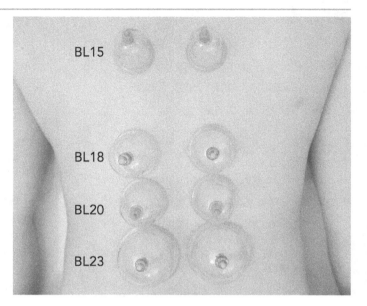

FATIGUE

A symptom of countless diseases, fatigue can cause a lack of physical strength, mental acuity, and motivation; sleepiness; exhaustion; poor concentration; poor memory; or inability to do the simplest things. For most people, it only happens occasionally when they don't get enough sleep, work too much, or are sick. However, others suffer for months and even years. Endocrine diseases (hypothyroidism, adrenal fatigue), cardiovascular diseases (anemia, heart failure), neuromuscular diseases (Parkinson's disease, multiple sclerosis), sleep disorders, mental illness, pain, infections, and medications can all cause fatigue. Since there are so many causes, it is important to get a proper diagnosis from your doctor to see where fatigue is coming from, especially if it's chronic or severe.

According to TCM, fatigue is usually caused by a deficiency of Qi, Blood, Yin, or Yang. Cupping can help strengthen back your organs to help produce more Qi, Blood, Yin, or Yang. Each organ is associated with an emotion, and prolonged exposure to these emotions can weaken its associated organ. The Lung is associated with grief, the Spleen is associated with overthinking, the Liver is associated with anger, the Kidney is associated with fear, and the Heart to overjoy. Cupping can help calm or ease your mind, as well as strengthen the organ that has been injured, relieving the fatigue.

CV12 *Zhong Wan–Central Stomach*

Location: On the anterior midline of the body, halfway between the sternum and umbilicus.

When to use: As a general point to tonify Qi, nourish the body, and improve digestion to get more nourishment from food.

Application: Use Weak to Medium Cupping twice a week for 10 to 15 minutes.

CV6 *Qi Hai–Sea of Qi*

Location: On the anterior midline of the body, around one thumb's length (or approximately 1.5 inches) below the umbilicus.

When to use: As a general point to tonify Qi and nourish the body.

Application: Use Weak to Medium Cupping twice a week for 10 to 15 minutes.

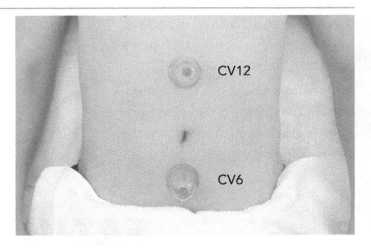

BL20 *Pi Shu–Spleen Shu*

Location: 1.5 inches on either side of the spinous process of the eleventh thoracic vertebra (T11).

When to use: General point to tonify Qi and nourish the body. Helps to improve digestion to get more nourishment from food.

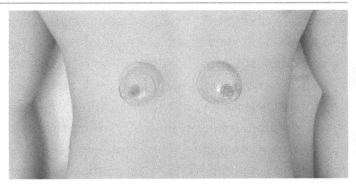

Application: Use Weak to Medium Cupping for 10 to 15 minutes twice a week.

ST36 *Zu San Li— Leg Three Miles*

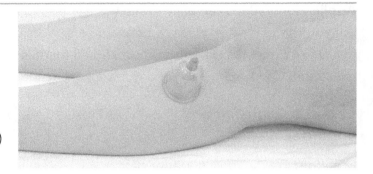

Location: Four fingers' width (or approximately 3 inches) below the inferior-lateral corner of the patella, and about a thumb's width (or 1 inch) lateral to the tibia (shinbone).

When to use: As a general point to tonify Qi, nourish the body, and improve digestion to get more nourishment from food.

Application: Use Weak to Medium Cupping twice a week for 10 to 15 minutes.

INSOMNIA

Insomnia is difficulty falling or staying asleep, waking up during the night with trouble going back to bed, waking up tired or too early, having restless sleep, or having dream-disturbed sleep. There are two kinds of insomnia: primary and secondary. Primary insomnia is not associated with any other disease or condition. Secondary insomnia is a direct consequence of another disease or health condition, such as asthma, depression, pain, heartburn, medication, or drug use. Insomnia can be acute or chronic.

According to TCM, sleep is governed by the Heart. The Heart can get agitated in a multitude of ways, leading to insomnia. If the Heart is not nourished properly, it can become agitated. The Heart can get stimulated by Heat, which can come from the environment through hot weather, or a hot room. Heat can also come from diet through spicy foods, greasy foods, caffeinated drinks, and alcohol. Cupping is good at clearing Heat from the body and calming the mind. The Heart can also get agitated by emotions, such as anger, stress, anxiety, and frustration. Cupping can help the Heart to relax.

GB20 *Feng Chi—Wind Pool*

Location: In the depression between the sternocleidomastoid muscle and the trapezius muscle, just at the base of the skull.

When to use: For any type of insomnia, especially if due to stress.

Application: GB20 is actually within the hairline, so a cup cannot be placed directly on it, but you can place it as close to the hairline as possible. Apply Weak or Medium Cupping for 10 to 15 minutes. Use stronger suction if there is more tension, and weaker suction for relaxation. Can be done every day if weaker suction is used.

GB21 *Jian Jing– Shoulder Well*

Location: On the most superior part of the shoulder, directly above the nipple, or halfway from the spine to the deltoid muscle.

When to use: For insomnia due to stress or neck and shoulder pain.

Application: Use Weak or Medium Cupping for 10 to 15 minutes. Use stronger suction if there is more tension, and weaker suction for relaxation. Can be done every day if weaker suction is used.

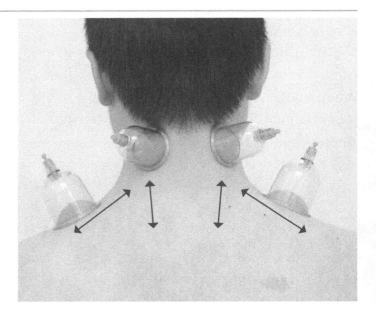

BL15 *Xin Shu–Heart Shu*

Location: 1.5 inches on either side of the spinous process of the fifth thoracic vertebra (T5).

When to use: For any mental symptoms, including insomnia, anxiety, stress, irritability, short-temperedness, or restlessness.

Application: Use Weak or Medium Cupping for 10 to 15 minutes. Use stronger suction if insomnia is due to stress, and weaker suction for relaxation. Can be done every day if weaker suction is used.

BL18 *Gan Shu–Liver Shu*

Location: 1.5 inches on either side of the spinous process of the ninth thoracic vertebra (T9).

When to use: For any mental symptoms, including insomnia, anxiety, stress, irritability, short-temperedness, restlessness, or depression. Especially useful if insomnia is due to emotions.

Application: Use Weak or Medium Cupping for 10 to 15 minutes. Use stronger suction if insomnia is due to stress, and weaker suction for relaxation. Can be done every day if weaker suction is used. Use slightly stronger suction or Moving Cupping up and down the back for general muscle tension.

BL20 *Pi Shu–Spleen Shu*

Location: 1.5 inches on either side of to the spinous process of the eleventh thoracic vertebra (T11).

When to use: For insomnia accompanied by fatigue.

Application: Use Weak or Medium Cupping for 10 to 15 minutes. Use stronger suction if insomnia is due to stress, and weaker suction for relaxation. Can be done every day if weaker suction is used.

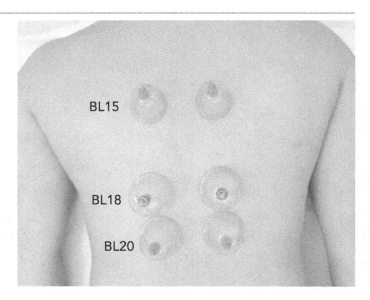

REFERENCES

Akhtar, Jamal, and M. Khalid Siddiqui. "Utility of Cupping Therapy Hijamat in Unani Medicine." *Indian Journal of Traditional Knowledge* 7, no. 4 (2008): 572–574.

Alban, Joseph. "Chinese Medicine for Acne." *Alban Acupuncture.* January 24, 2011. Retrieved March 22, 2012. http://albanacupuncture.com/blog/chinese-medicine-for-acne.

Al-Jauziyah, Qayyim. *Healing with the Medicine of the Prophet.* Lahore, Pakistan: Darussalam Publishers, 2003.

Cao, Huijian, Mei Han, et al. "An Overview of Systematic Reviews of Clinical Evidence for Cupping Therapy." *Journal of Traditional Chinese Medical Sciences* 2, no. 1 (2015): 3–10. doi: 10.1016/j.jtcms.2014.11.012.

Chirali, Ilkay. *Traditional Chinese Medicine Cupping Therapy.* London: Churchhill Livingstone Elsevier Ltd., 2014.

Cui, Shuai and Jin Cui. "Progress of Researches on the Mechanism of Cupping Therapy." *Zhen Ci Yan Jiu (Acuptuncture Research)* 37, no. 6 (2012): 506–10.

"Effective Home Remedies for Pimples and Acne Vulgaris." ChineseMedicineAdvisor.com. Retrieved March 26, 2012, http://www.chinesemedicineadvisor.com/home-remedies-for-pimples.html.

Emerich, Markus, Hans-Willi Clement, et al. "Mode of Action of Cupping—Local Metabolism and Pain Thresholds in Neck Pain Patients and Healthy Subjects." *Complementary Therapies in Medicine* 22, no. 1 (2014): 148–158. doi: 10.1016/j.ctim.2013.12.013.

Epstein, J. "The Therapeutic Value of Cupping." *New York Medical Journal* 112 (1920): 584–585.

Hanninen, Osmo, and Tuula Vaskilampi. "Cupping as a Part of Living Finnish Traditional Healing. A Remedy against Pain." *Acupuncture & Electro-Therapeutics Research* 7, no. 1 (1982): 39–50. doi: 10.3727/036012982816952161.

Harper, Donald John. *Early Chinese Medical Literature: The Mawangdui Medical Manuscripts.* London: Kegan Paul International, 1998.

Lange, Susan. "Acne and Pimples: Top 7 Factors to Healing Acne, Pimples & Other Skin Conditions with Chinese Medicine." *Meridian Holistic Health.* March 11, 2009. Retrieved

March 26, 2012. http://meridianholistic.com/healthyliving/acne-and-pimples-top-7-factors-to-healing-acne-pimples-other-skin-conditions-with-chinese-medicine

Lee, Myeong Soo, Jong-In Kim, et al. "Is Cupping an Effective Treatment? An Overview of Systematic Reviews." *Journal of Acupuncture and Meridian Studies* 4, no. 1 (2011): 1-4. doi: 10.1016/S2005-2901(11)60001-0.

Mehta, Piyush, and Vividha Dhapte. "Cupping Therapy: A Prudent Remedy for a Plethora of Medical Ailments." *Journal of Traditional and Complementary Medicine* 5, no. 3 (2015): 127–134. doi: 10.1016/j.jtcme.2014.11.036.

Nimrouzi, Majid, Ali Mahbodi et al. "Hijama in Traditional Persian Medicine: Risks and Benefits." *Journal of Evidence-Based Integrative Medicine* 19, no. 2 (2014): 128–136. doi: 10.117/2156587214524578.

Rozenfeld, Evgeni, and Leonid Kalichman. "New Is the Well-Forgotten Old: The Use of Dry Cupping in Musculoskeletal Medicine." *Journal of Bodywork & Movement Therapies* 20, no. 1 (January 2016): 173–178. doi: 10.1016/j.jbmt.2015.11.009.

Schulte, E.. "Complementary Therapies: Acupuncture: Where East Meets West." *Research Nursing* 59, no. 10 (1996): 55–57.

Shen Herbal Pharmacy. "Chinese Medicine and Herbs for Acne." Retrieved March 26, 2012. http://www.drshen.com/herbsforacne.htm.

"Spot Positions, Acne Locations and Chinese Face Mapping." SayWhyDoI.com. August 19, 2011. Retrieved March 26, 2012. http://www.saywhydoi.com/spot-positions-acne-locations-and-chinese-face-mapping.

Tham, L. M., H. P. Lee, et al. "Cupping: From a Biomechanical Perspective." *Journal of Biomechanics* 39, no. 12 (2006): 2183–93. doi: 10.1016/j.jbiomech.2005.06.027.

Turk, J. L. and Elizabeth Allen. "Bleeding and Cupping." *Annals of The Royal College of Surgeons of England* 65, no. 2 (1983): 128–133.

"What Causes Acne." Skinacea. January 2, 2012. Retrieved March 22, 2012. http://www.skinacea.com/acne/acne-causes.html.

Yoo, Simon, and Francisco Tausk. "Cupping: East Meets West." *International Journal of Dermatology* 43, no. 9 (2004): 664–665. doi: 10.1111/j.1365-4632.2004.02224.x.

INDEX

ACKNOWLEDGMENTS

I would like to thank my parents, Benny and Anne Choi, for being good role models of what a kind and compassionate person should be. Thank you for your support—financially, physically, and emotionally—through my many years of schooling. I wouldn't be where I am now without your support and guidance. I would also like to thank my sister, Joanna Choi, for helping shape me into who I am today.

I would also like to thank Mary Wu, owner of the Toronto School of Traditional Chinese Medicine, for being the reason I am in TCM today. Thank you for your hard work in promoting and advocating TCM in Ontario and in Canada. Thank you for all your long days and nights teaching and running the school. Thank you for seeing the potential in me and giving me the opportunity to teach acupuncture and TCM.

Thanks to Linda Tang and Richard Kwan for being my TCM mentors. You have not only taught me the way to be a good practitioner, but also showed me how to be passionate about this medicine, and how to show compassion to my patients.

I would like to thank Enza Ierullo, owner of Acupuncture and Integrative Medicine Academy, for seeing the potential in me and helping me to advance in the field of TCM education. Your endless toil for the school in the midst of everything going on is an inspiration to me.

Thank you to Jocelyn Choi for connecting me to Ulysses Press, so that I can have this opportunity to share my experience and help more people that I would never have been able to reach.

Thank you William Shin for the wonderful photos. Thank you Daniel Cheung and Jessica Chin for being the models for my book.

Lastly, I would like to thank my better half for supporting me, and encouraging me through the writing of the book. I couldn't have done it without you.

I would like to dedicate this book to our God and Saviour, Jesus Christ, my Rock and my Redeemer.

ABOUT THE AUTHOR

Kenneth Choi is a Registered Acupuncturist as well as a Registered Traditional Chinese Medicine Practitioner in Canada. He is a member of the College of Traditional Chinese Medicine Practitioners and Acupuncturists of Ontario.

Kenneth graduated from University of Toronto with his Honors Bachelor of Science in Human Biology, specializing in Genes, Genetics, and Biotechnology. He then went on to graduate from McGill University with his Masters of Science in Biotechnology. He received his Chinese Medicine training from the Toronto School of Traditional Chinese Medicine in Toronto, Canada, where he graduated with the 4-Year Advanced Traditional Chinese Medicine diploma.

He has been teaching Acupuncture and Chinese Herbology for 5 years at the Toronto School of Traditional Chinese Medicine and at the Academy and Integrative Medicine Academy. He is currently the Director of the Acupuncture Program and Chinese Herbology Program at the Acupuncture and Integrative Medicine Academy in Toronto, Ontario, Canada. Kenneth also practices Acupuncture and Chinese Herbology at his clinic, Richmond Hill Acupuncture and Natural Therapy Clinic, in Richmond Hill, Ontario.